Mayim's
VEGAN TABLE

Mayim's
VEGAN TABLE

More Than 100 Great-Tasting and Healthy Recipes from My Family to Yours

Mayim Bialik

with Dr. Jay Gordon

Da Capo

LIFE
LONG

A Member of the Perseus Books Group

Published by Da Capo Press
A Member of the Perseus Books Group
www.dacapopress.com

Library of Congress Cataloging-in-Publication Data is available for this book.
ISBN 978-0-7382-1704-8 (paperback)
ISBN 978-0-7382-1705-5 (e-book)

Da Capo Press books are available at special discounts for bulk purchases in the U.S. by corporations, institutions, and other organizations. For more information, please contact the Special Markets Department at the Perseus Books Group, 2300 Chestnut Street, Suite 200, Philadelphia, PA, 19103, or call (800) 810-4145, ext. 5000, or e-mail special .markets@perseusbooks.com.

Editorial production by *Marra*thon Production Services. www.marrathon.net

Book design by Jane Raese
Set in 10-point Linoletter Medium

FIRST DA CAPO PRESS EDITION 2014
10 9 8 7 6 5 4 3 2 1

For my *zeis* children, Miles Roosevelt and Frederick Heschel
Tsurris mit yoykh iz gringer vi tsurris on yoykh—
Troubles with soup is easier than troubles without soup

You have changed my life immeasurably, and as I prepare food for you,
my prayer is that I can help you thrive inside and out.
I love being your mother and I love cooking for you.

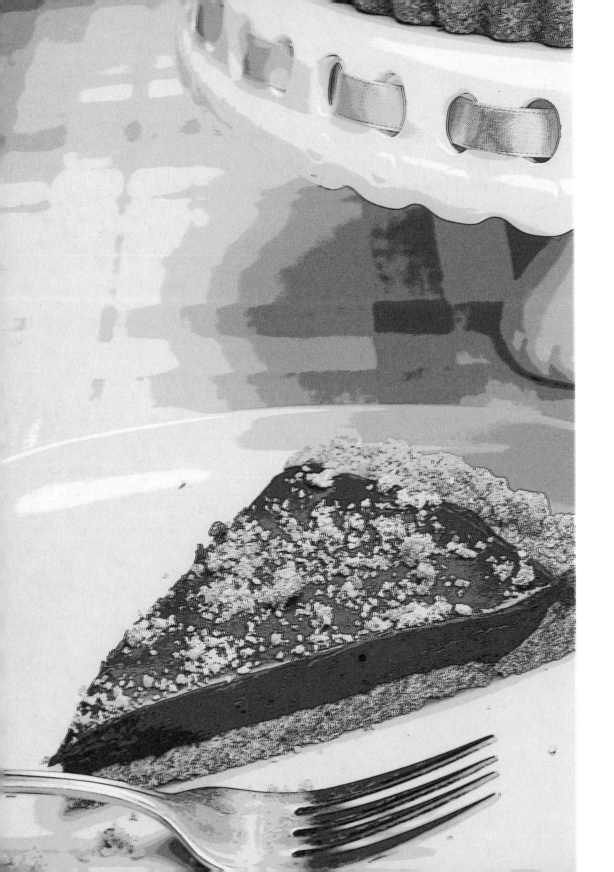

Contents

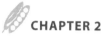
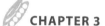
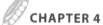
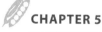

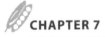

CHAPTER 7

Snacks, Sauces, and Dips 107

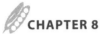

CHAPTER 8

Veggies and Sides 123

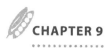
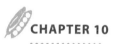
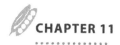

CHAPTER 1

Who Are We and Why Are We Telling You What to Eat?

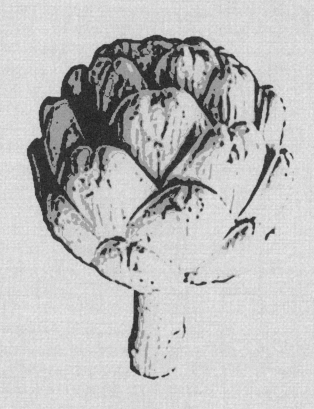

The past few years have been monumental for those passionate about plant-based eating. The word *vegan* used to have a lot of baggage attached to it and suggested certain stereotypes. Fortunately for the vegan and nonvegan alike, however, there has been a pronounced move for all of us to incorporate more plant-based foods into our diets to combat the obesity epidemic and help us live longer and healthier lives. This includes general recommendations, such as eating more fruit, more vegetables, more whole grains, fewer processed foods, and fewer salty and fatty foods. Regardless of whether you embrace a plant-based, omnivorous, or carnivorous diet, it is now universally accepted that everyone would benefit from a diet of plant-based foods.

You may have picked up this book because you want to learn more about plant-based choices for your family and how they can impact your family's health and well-being. Maybe you just want a change from what you've been eating so you can have more energy and know that you are eating things that are natural and good. And maybe you're curious about whether a plant-based philosophy and lifestyle could ever satisfy your palate.

The authors of the book you hold in your hands weren't raised vegan, and our journeys to veganism are as different as we are. Dr. Jay is a pediatrician, pediatric nutritionist, and international board-certified lactation consultant who has been helping families achieve happy and wholesome living for over thirty years. He has been a vegan for almost forty years and eats whole foods almost exclusively, no preservatives, and almost no sugars. Dr. Jay grew up in and went to medical school in Wisconsin, where he took care of people who had made some pretty bad nutritional decisions. (Have you ever been to a movie theater in Wisconsin? They serve deep-fried cheese balls!) In his last year of medical school, after treating way too many overweight people who had heart disease and cancer, he became a chocolate-chip-cookie-grilled-cheese-sandwich-french-fry-potato-chip vegetarian for a number of years. ("That doughnut doesn't have any meat in it, does it?!") Although there wasn't a specific "aha!" moment, he did begin a gradual transition to soy cheese and other, better alternatives. Over time, he realized that eating "real" foods—those that are unprocessed and as close to "whole" as possible—was better still. Dr. Jay's personal eating habits are *still* evolving, changing, improving.

Besides being an Emmy-nominated actress, author, and a trained neuroscientist, Mayim is the mother of two sons who have been raised entirely vegan. However, Mayim's journey to veganism involved years of cutting back on certain foods before cutting them out entirely. What started as eliminating dairy for health reasons and because of her son's sensitivity to dairy during breastfeeding grew to an overhaul of eating and thinking patterns. Mayim now considers herself a vegan motivated by concerns for her health and that of her family, environmental considerations about the impact of animals raised for food, and ethical consideration as well. Her transition from a vegetarian college student to an almost vegan mom to a now entirely vegan mom involved a strong need for "fun foods"—foods that can please finicky toddler palates, and a lifestyle that is not expensive, time consuming, or only available if there are vegan restaurants around. Mayim's life is that of a working mom with a practical and down-to-earth sensibility; she doesn't belong to an exclusive community of vegans who can't eat out or let their kids go to other kids' houses for fear they would eat a slice of cheese.

Ultimately, we don't expect anyone to pick up this book and become an "instant vegan" but instead to become a more thoughtful eater and "feeder" of children and families. Slow but steady is just fine with us. It's what we've done and continue to do. And if you already do practice a plant-based diet, we hope you'll enjoy our nutritional guidance and delicious recipes.

Throughout the chapters of this book, we will take on the most common misconceptions and myths about vegans, veganism, and plant-based eating—especially when it comes to nutrition and feeding our families. Our hope is to not hide behind such clichés as "Everyone should be vegan!," "It's easy to be vegan!," and "Your life will be a million times better if you just do everything we say!" We know that's not going to work for most people. What we have decided to do is be up front about what we assume you are thinking, because we have thought it all ourselves! We hope to clarify some of these misconceptions and, if nothing else, to put some delicious information on your plate so that you can best decide what works for you and your family. And we'll help you put it all into action with over 100 easy recipes that have been tested on kids and adults.

Who Is Vegan?

Vegans are a diverse crowd and there's a lot of variability in nutritional, ethical, and lifestyle choices. Some vegans are 100 percent vegan right down to their nonleather shoes and faux leather belts. Other people eat vegan for health reasons but have no ethical or environmental considerations that influence their decision to be vegan. Mike Tyson has stopped biting ears and has gone vegan. Russell Simmons and Ellen DeGeneres: vegan, too. Even Bill Clinton has a mostly vegan diet. So, whatever your image of a vegan may be, start picturing yourself and those you love. Because we think you're going to love it.

There are people who choose vegan meals whenever there is any option to do so, but know that there may be meals served to them from time to time that may contain a possible dairy or egg ingredient. These people express that the intent of eating and living completely vegan is crucially important to them and that the practical aspects of going from 99 to 100 percent vegan eating are often the most difficult.

We have made the decision to be 100 percent vegan. What we hope to do here is give you some of the basics of nutrition, talk about where your food comes from, and offer you options so you can decide for yourself what will work for your family. The subtleties of politics, the environment, and the ethical and humane considerations of the usage of animals for food and clothing may be things you're already aware of, may take much longer for you to learn about, or may never appeal to you. The bottom line: only you know what will work for your family and at what pace changes may be incorporated. The changes we suggest, such as eating more whole foods, more fruits and vegetables, and fewer processed foods, have been universally recommended for years by leading medical health authorities. We care less about what you call yourself and more that you get useful information and delicious recipes from us.

But Does It Taste Good?

We'd like to set the record straight that first and foremost we, Mayim and Dr. Jay, love food. (We *really love food.*) It used to be that you had to choose between "good" food and healthy food.

That's not so anymore! Even the most dedicatedly vegan families we know eat and enjoy great food, and there are tons of fast, easy, inexpensive ways to do that.

Second, it is not our intention for you or your kids to never have another french fry.

We don't want to deprive you—and french fries happen. But we're letting kids know that there are foods that we're not going out and getting as a routine food. You get into real trouble if the once-in-a-while foods become regular ones. This book is full of rich and sometimes delightfully greasy foods that will satisfy you and your children, but because you are preparing them, you'll naturally moderate how often you enjoy them. And as for french fries? Give your kids a dry paper towel to squeeze because we've got a great recipe on PAGE 135 for OVEN-BAKED FRIES!

Although the ease with which you can order "anything" at restaurants, in foreign countries, and at cocktail parties will change if your diet is entirely plant-based, being plant-based isn't a punishment. It's a commitment to health and well-being that necessitates being open to a world of new tastes and textures and flavors.

Third, most people already enjoy many foods that they don't realize are vegan or easily veganized. Almost all store-bought boxed pastas are egg-free. Asian food typically uses no dairy, and Indian cuisine tends to feature tons of vegetables and a host of sauces and flavors of dishes that don't have any meat, provided you skip the ghee and yogurt these recipes sometimes use. Bean-based chilis and stews are easily vegan. If you avoid the cheese, Mexican and South American food is full of vegetables and beans and grains that also do not require meat to be enjoyable. Besides featuring some of the best vegan foods ever (falafel, hummus, tahini), Mediterranean food consists of many delicious salads made of peppers, eggplant, carrots, cabbage, rice, and fantastic spices, all without dairy or meat. In short: great food awaits you!

The recipes in this book are Dr. Jay–approved and come from Mayim's own kitchen, with a handful of Dr. Jay's favorites thrown in there as well. Our families have different ranges of ages, and we will cover a little bit of everything from great foods for picky toddlers to meals for seemingly insatiable teenagers and their seemingly unimpressable gourmet-palate parents, too. We have selected recipes that have been known to please even the most skeptical carnivores. Very few of these recipes seek to mimic meat or dairy; they are the meals that we make most frequently for our families and for our vegan and nonvegan friends alike, which are met with the most enthusiastic responses and requests for "more, please!"

Plant-based eating comes about for a lot of reasons, and there's no "right" way to start incorporating more fruits, vegetables, and grains into your and your family's diet. You can change slowly, and in a way that works for your family. Our plant-based diets are really excellent and tasty and yours can be, too. It's about learning to build a diet on simple whole foods, and then it's about embracing a new kind of cuisine that includes all of the tastes and textures and feelings of fun and pleasure we all associate with wonderful food.

It's about complex flavors, rich hearty soups, simple and awe-inspiring sandwiches, and greens that your salad-phobic friends won't run screaming from. It's about not missing out just because you are choosing to be a person who doesn't eat meat or dairy. And—yes!—it's about those decadent pies and cakes and cookies and truffles, too! It's learning what you can have, when you can have it, and learning to love it, rather than living your life according to what you think you "can't" have.

DR. JAY: Ear infection? Rash that won't go away? Try cutting out all dairy for three weeks. See what happens. My experience says you'll see a difference. What have you got to lose?

If That's Not Enough to Convince You

We save the nutritional aspects of veganism for Chapter 2, where we really delve into the vegan diet and discuss healthy choices that will work best for your needs. Here are some of the health, environmental, and ethical aspects of a vegan lifestyle.

Health

The consumption of animal products has been associated with and confirmed to be responsible for numerous cancers, cardiovascular problems, and obesity. Sometimes it's hard to explain to kids (and adults!) that kids who are eating junk and look just as tall and strong as kids who don't, aren't as healthy as they appear! Dr. Jay explains, "They might look the same on the outside. They might look and feel the same for a while. But a high-fat, high-sugar diet is going to catch up with them." As he tells his patients, "If you're going to build a nice house, are you going to build it with junky wood and junky bricks or are you going to get the very best stuff? And if you're building healthy soccer players, or dancers, or guitarists, would you want to build them out of junky food or the best food?" Kids always know the right answer.

Chronic ear infections, sore throats, allergies, sinus infections, stomach-aches, gastrointestinal troubles ranging from mild to severe, acne and rashes, in addition to the "big" health problems—there is a host of food-associated sensitivities that many of us are not told can be reduced or eliminated with dietary changes. It's not only the research that backs us up; we've seen firsthand startling changes in these types of problems in our very own families and among our broader circle of friends and patients, simply from shifting to more plant-based diets.

More vegan choices mean stronger bones, stronger muscles, and kids who get sick less often. Choosing not to eat meat and dairy means you are promoting great health and fitness on a daily basis and avoiding lifelong medical problems. For your health, your children's health, and the health of the nation and the world, that's simply the truth.

Environment and Ethics

Bill Maher once quipped, "The business of raising animals for food causes about 40 percent more global warming than all cars, trucks, and planes combined. If you care about the planet, it's actually better to eat a salad in a Hummer than a cheeseburger in a Prius." And if that's not enough, it takes 12 pounds of grain and 2,500 gallons of water to create a single pound of beef. We literally use more resources to grow food for the animals we eat than

I'M GOING TO HAVE TO EMPTY MY BANK ACCOUNT TO EAT THIS WAY, RIGHT?

Here's the lowdown: plant-based eating and living is for people of all socio-economic backgrounds. It isn't necessarily expensive—if you plan it out. It is true that you may find yourself buying more produce than before, and if you choose to buy organic, you'll want to figure out a simple budget for that. It also helps to know which fruits and veggies gather the most pesticides from the earth where they are grown. Buying pesticide-free foods is very important when you're feeding children because their rapidly growing brain and body might be more susceptible to injury from the chemicals in conventionally grown foods. The problem with pesticides is that children, pound for pound, eat more apple slices and blueberries than adults do. This means that if a certain amount of pesticide has been deemed safe for a 150-pound adult, it probably isn't safe for a 35-pound child. Very few adults focus with the fervor of toddlers on one food type. When children eat a basket of blueberries in a sitting, they're ingesting, pound for pound, more poison in their food during the years when they have the least tolerance.

Check out the "Dirty Dozen and Clean Fifteen" box on PAGE 50. It'll help you decide which foods to buy organic. That's what works for a lot of families. To rephrase a medical cliché, if you think eating organic is expensive, try pricing poor health and illness.

Many vegan families tend to eat simply a lot of the time, with staples of their diet consisting of bulk items, such as beans and grains and rice and quinoa. Many of us choose to save resources for organic items and specialty items that cost more than animal-based alternatives and also budget in other ways, such as eliminating expensive and often unnecessary cleaning products, reducing the use of paper products, and buying gently used clothing, toys, and books rather than purchasing everything new so that there is money left for the foods we want to buy organic. (You may not think that we practice these methods ourselves, but we do!)

There is no "right" way to figure any of this out; it's not easy to make those decisions, but eating and living this way can be done within a budget.

to feed the hungry in our cities, our country, our world. It doesn't have to be that way.

Not all vegans choose to be vegan because of ethical considerations. For those of us who do, here are some of the things we think about. We're not here to gross anyone out—there are plenty of other resources showing what it's like for workers and animals in factory farms that will do that. We simply want to lay out the basic ethical issues and let you decide how much you want to learn beyond this very brief summary.

Meat from animals raised in factories is recalled frequently because the animals are raised in filthy conditions. They're crowded together and have to be given antibiotics to prevent the diseases they spread to one another. (Consequently, these antibiotics are in our food supply as well and contribute to antibiotic resistance and health problems for us.)

In nature, chickens lay a few eggs a day and cows only produce milk when they are nursing a calf, typically once a year. Hormone injections and artificial boosting of these animals' normal physiology is how we get the amounts of dairy and eggs needed for a factory to be considered "successful and productive." Grass-fed farms and such may have better living conditions when they are well regulated, but the issue of slaughter technique and considerations for animal welfare is still very troublesome and, in many cases, quite disturbing even to the most happy meat eater.

Factory workers are paid notoriously poor wages and are not treated humanely themselves. If we continue to support industries that treat humans and animals in cruel and careless ways, then we become part of a very real problem our children will inherit.

There's much more information available on health, environmental, and ethical concerns. We found the documentary *Food, Inc.* to be really informative; you'll find more suggestions for further information in the Resources section in the back of the book. In the next chapter, we'll tackle nutrition and structuring the vegan diet. Then, let's set the table for fun food, healthy and wholesome choices, and decadent and delicious reminders that plant-based is anything but boring.

We want you to love what you eat and eat what you love. Let's do it.

THIS IS TOO TIME CONSUMING AND OVERWHELMING!
I'M TOO BUSY FOR THIS!

This is an understandable concern, and it's one we have been through, too. Two things helped as we struggled with this. First, we needed to admit once and for all that we didn't want to eat as many processed foods, animal products, sugar, salt, and preservatives anymore. It's not good for the body, especially a growing body.

The second thing that helped us commit to being open to change was to hear the following: once you commit to making a change, no matter how small, you will see that it is not any harder, more time consuming, or more labor intensive to eat and cook and live this way. Partly, this will be because you understand deeply the principles of health and nutrition to the extent that we will present them. And partly, it's because you will find a rhythm. You will cook and freeze things. You will discover easy fast snacks and favorite items for you and your kids, and your palate will change. You and your kids will learn over time to love an apple and a handful of almonds as a snack. We can and will be satisfied with wholesome plant-based foods.

Once you make small changes, it's actually going to be not that different from where you are now. But it will be healthier and tastier. How's that for a trade-off?

Have ever heard the quote, "Be kind to your knees. You'll miss them when they're gone"? Well, if your kids knew how important it is to eat well now and to age gracefully into their teens, and to be stronger and healthier when they're twenty or thirty or forty or fifty, there wouldn't be any arguments. They don't know. We know. Your kids are going to be happy that we did this for them now while they're young and can't understand. Your efforts are worth it.

CHAPTER 2

Is Plant-Based Eating
Really Better for Us?
Nutritional Choices

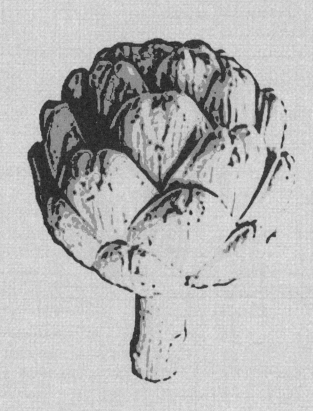

When we tell people we are vegan, one of the first things we tend to hear back is something along the lines of, "But is that really healthy?" And, "But where do you get your protein?" Out-of-date myths about vegans being malnourished, lacking adequate calcium and protein, suffering from vitamin B_{12} deficiency, and having a pale and sickly appearance abound. Significant literature has already tackled some of the most persuasive arguments and scientifically tested and proven benefits to a vegan diet, and we have listed in the Resources section some of the most reliable books that handle this matter. What we want to do is talk to you about why a plant-based diet works really well and the problems that occur when you and your children eat in other ways.

In the next section, we'll talk about what's wrong and unscientific about how many of us were raised to think about food. What's problematic about milk and cheese and eggs, from a nutritional perspective? What about beef, chicken, or fish? And what are some alternatives that take into consideration not just taste but nutrition as well? We'll cover it all.

From a purely medical point of view, the majority of doctors and other experts can tell you that eating too much red meat and cheese is bad for you and your family. Milk is allergenic and very few children are healthier because they drink milk. The CDC's (Centers for Disease Control) most recent report named chicken as causing the largest proportion of deaths from food-borne illness.[1] No wonder. Most chickens are raised with enough antibiotics and other chemicals to give pause to any parent or scientist. Fish are contaminated because we have treated our waterways so badly. Let's get into some more specifics.

Milk: It Does a Body

The vast majority of Americans feel that it's important to drink milk throughout their lives. If your baby or child happens to weigh in at the low end of the growth chart at the pediatrician, many well-meaning but under-informed doctors prescribe whole milk. There is an almost universally accepted notion that whole fat milk builds better bodies and brains. Milk is, indeed, a significant source of protein and calcium, and as many die-hard milk drinkers will tell you, they like getting all of that protein and calcium in one simple glass rather than having to get it from other food sources or supplements.

What's true is that cow's milk is specifically designed to efficiently grow . . . a baby cow. Cows have huge bodies and comparatively small brains, walk within hours of birth, mature within months, and die within a short number of years. There's simply no scientific basis for feeding cow's milk to human children. None. Dr. Jay asks his young patients, "Are you a cow? Only cows drink cow's milk! Are you a yak? Only yaks drink yak's milk!" They get the idea.

The American Academy of Pediatrics is very clear that a child should have human milk for his or her entire first year. And it has recently joined every other reputable expert group in recommending that period of time as a minimum, not an endpoint. Water is the best weaning beverage for babies over a year of age.

Milk also can increase the tendency for tonsillitis, runny stuffy noses, and ear infections. Milk from another species is highly immunogenic, which means that it triggers an allergic immune response that may look like anything from hives to diarrhea. An adverse reaction to milk can include bloating, indigestion, and a variety of gastrointestinal problems that are consistent with the fact that approximately 25 percent of Caucasians, 90 percent of Asian Americans, and 75

DR. JAY: I tell kids that the dairy industry spends hundreds of millions of dollars each year to convince you that milk is good for you.[4] If milk were good for you, the dairy industry wouldn't have to spend hundreds of millions of dollars to convince you of that—nobody is spending more than a buck ninety-eight to convince you that broccoli is good for you! You know that broccoli is good for you. All this money is being spent on selling milk and cheese because they're ultimately not good for your health, and it's trying to counter real science with fake mustaches and the "goal" to have a body like David Beckham,[5] which most of us can never have, no matter how hard we work at it.

percent of Mexican Americans, Native Americans, Eastern European Jews, and African Americans lack the enzyme for digesting lactose and are lactose intolerant and/or have adverse reactions to milk.[2]

Milk has been linked to prostate cancer and ovarian cancer as well.[3] It is also associated with obesity and cardiovascular disease. Babies who drink cow's milk in the first year of life are much more likely to be anemic and this anemia can lead to school-age learning disabilities.[6] Put plainly, animal-based milk has very few nutritional benefits that outweigh the health challenges it presents. How to obtain enough calcium is often the biggest question, but there are plenty of great nondairy sources. If you're worried about calcium, don't be.

Alternatives

While it is true that substitute, nondairy, milks may never taste the same as cow's milk when they are compared glass to glass, the world of nondairy milks can change the way you eat cereal, the way you bake, and the way you make cream sauces and dressings. The most common milk substitutes are almond milk, rice milk, and soy milk, all of which contain calcium and protein,

> **DR. JAY:** Add a little bit of your alternative milk at a time, maybe just a couple of teaspoons to start. No hurry. Over time you will have made the change and hardly noticed the difference. This goes for all the ways you'll transition to a vegan diet. Do it gradually. Adding and deleting. Take. Your. Time.

and all of which are available vitamin D fortified. Each has slightly different texture, sugar content, and taste, and there is no real rhyme or reason as to when to use which. It depends on what tastes best to you, and while some people report better success making vegan cream sauces out of "heavier" milks, such as soy or almond, it really is up to you to decide which tastes and feels the best. Also, if you are watching your fat or sugar intake, which Dr. Jay says we all should be, you will want to compare the nutritional content of various milks to see which suits your needs. Admittedly, it takes anywhere from a few weeks to a few months to fully shift your palate from cow's milk to a nondairy milk, but every vegan we know reports that after a little while, there is no more comparing. There is simply the enjoyment of eating and making recipes that you thought you couldn't without cow's milk!

You can find calcium in so many places. Broccoli is an excellent source of calcium. It contains about the same amount as milk, ounce for ounce. When a child is old enough to eat unprocessed soy, 1.5 ounces of tofu will provide the same amount of calcium as a glass of skim milk. Unconvinced about the benefits of soy? Studies show that women who consume soy are less likely to develop breast cancer.

FOOD	AMOUNT	CALCIUM (MG)
Blackstrap molasses	2 tablespoons	400
Collard greens, cooked	1 cup	357
Other plant milks, calcium-fortified	8 ounces	300–500
Tofu, processed with calcium sulfate	4 ounces	200–420
Calcium-fortified orange juice	8 ounces	350
Soy or rice milk, commercial, calcium-fortified, plain	8 ounces	200–300
Commercial soy yogurt, plain	6 ounces	300
Turnip greens, cooked	1 cup	249
Tofu, processed with nigari	4 ounces	130–400
Tempeh	1 cup	184
Kale, cooked	1 cup	179
Soybeans, cooked	1 cup	175
Bok choy, cooked	1 cup	158
Mustard greens, cooked	1 cup	152
Okra, cooked	1 cup	135
Tahini	2 tablespoons	128
Navy beans, cooked	1 cup	126
Almond butter	2 tablespoons	111
Almonds, whole	¼ cup	94
Broccoli, cooked	1 cup	62

Source: http://www.vrg.org/nutrition/calcium.php

They may need to consume it early in their life when breast tissue is still forming—all the more reason to start feeding it to your children now.

Most of the dark green leafy vegetables provide calcium, and there are smaller but still important amounts in many fruits, vegetables, nuts, grains, and seeds. Orange juice and cereals are available calcium-fortified, as are many nut and rice milks (as mentioned earlier). Lots of kids find dark greens too strong but you can finely chop the greens and add them to less strong-tasting greens, such as spinach, or in a vegetable soup. Green smoothies are great options, too—with fruit, nut milks, and/or nut butters, kids won't even taste the greens. Sesame seeds are also a good source of calcium and you can add them to mashed potatoes or sprinkle them on salads. Sesame butter can be used in place of peanut butter. If you're still concerned about calcium intake, you can buy calcium supplements wherever vitamins are sold. The chart on page 15 shows fantastic foods that are rich in calcium.[7] We think you'll find enough great choices here for your family if you want to get calcium from nonanimal sources!

Chuck the Cheese

Like milk, cheese is a concentrated source of calcium and protein. And like milk, cheese has a ton of fat (it's one of the highest-fat foods) and calories: 300 calories of cheese fits in the palm of your hand, but to get 300 calories of broccoli, you'd need a basket!

According to Michael Moss in *Salt, Sugar, Fat*, Americans eat 33 pounds of cheese and cheese products per year, per person—which is triple the consumption rate of the 1970s. Let's face it: cheese is very addictive because it's very salty and kids love the strong taste. Adults find it pretty tasty, too. Once you learn to like cheese, you never really learn to "unlike" it and it's hard to make it just a "fun" or some-

DR. JAY: If I could remove cheese and apple juice from every kid's diet, I think I could knock out the diagnosis of ADHD and obesity all at once! Zero cheese might not be very realistic for many kids, but we sure as heck should stop serving cheese and pepperoni pizza at every birthday party.

times food. Kids love cheese and many of them would always rather eat cheese than anything else. Most adults (us included) would also rather eat cheese than anything else!

Low-fat cheese is still one of the highest-fat foods in the supermarket. Talking about low-fat cheese is like talking about the smallest bull elephant at the zoo. It's still a pretty big animal. And sodium? One popular brand of organic mozzarella string cheese has 200 mg of sodium per stick of cheese and another brand of string cheese sticks has 190 mg of sodium per stick. A stick of cheese and another stick, and before you know it, you've acquired a really poor eating habit. Parents who tell their kids they can't have any cake at a party until they finish their pizza have really missed the boat. Simple statement: nobody is healthier because they eat cheese. And no one should smile when they say cheese, either!

As with dairy, it turns out that calcium is a moot point. There are so many calcium-rich vegan foods. And if you're concerned about protein, we'll talk about that shortly!

Alternatives

There are plenty of other sources of protein, but a lot of times what people miss about cheese is, well, its salty strong, familiar taste. While finding substitute vegan cheeses can be more complicated, the past few years alone have seen a phenomenal increase in a complex and exciting variety of cheese alternatives. Many "vegetarian" cheeses contain casein, a milk protein that makes them not okay for vegans. Gourmet vegan restaurants have been touting vegan goat cheese and nacho cheese for years, but it was considered a very rigorous and difficult set of recipes to try and master at home.

Nowadays, vegan cheeses, such as Daiya, are available in the supermarket and have transformed the vegan landscape. Daiya's non-soy-based excellence makes it ideal for pizza, cheese sauces, and anything that involves melted cheese, such as grilled cheese or quesadillas. Daiya also has a few flavors of Havarti, pepper jack, and provolone that have an incredible texture and taste. Other independent brands of vegan cheese are also making their way into supermarkets. While such store-bought cheeses as these are not considered "whole foods" and should be eaten sparingly because they contain fillers and preservatives—as do all store-bought cheeses—they have varying nutritional properties, depending on if they are soy based, tapioca based, or nut based. As we will discuss in Chapter 3, these should be considered "fun foods" and should not be considered the mainstay of your vegan diet, nor a source of calcium or protein equivalent to animal-based cheeses. (There are plenty of other nonanimal sources of both of these crucial nutrients.)

There are tons of easy and delicious ways to make cheese substitutes that can be spread on crackers, used as crudités for veggies , and even melted over tortilla chips for homemade nachos. In addition, artisan vegan cheese is now a "hot" arena, with cashew-based chèvre, buffalo mozzarella, and swiss appearing on market shelves and in homes of brave vegans prepared to put some time and effort into straining soy yogurt and soaking cashews for the reward of vegan artisanal cheese. Other, more basic nut-cheese recipes can be easily made at home, and you'll find some of those recipes in Chapter 9. These nut-based cheeses are a wonderful source of fat, protein, and a variety of vitamins and minerals. We like to think of them as creative and yummy ways to enjoy the wonderful world of nuts!

Butter and Ice Cream

Not a lot of people will tout dairy butter for its nutritional profile or health benefits. For most folks, it's all about the taste. For all of the reasons that the manufacture and consumption of milk and cheese is problematic, butter and ice cream are, too.

Vegan alternatives to butter exist that are great for cooking, baking, sautés, and even spreading on a piece of toast. Of course, vegan spreads don't taste exactly the same as butter—Mayim thinks they taste even better! But your taste buds will adjust faster than you think. You will also learn to love other spreads made of fruit and nuts and other yummy, rich-tasting things.

As for ice cream, there are so many alternatives to ice cream that range from frozen fruits run through a blender when a sweet craving hits, to store-bought and homemade nondairy ice creams using a variety of bases, the most popular of which are soy, almond, rice, and coconut milk. Children can enjoy (in reasonable amounts, mind you!) vegan ice-cream sandwiches, chocolate-covered ice-cream balls, chocolate chip cookie dough ice cream, ice cream pops, and more. Being vegan does not mean forgoing; it means making specific choices and being creative in the process!

Eggs (They're Not All They're Cracked Up to Be)

Eggs are an example of a food that packs a protein punch and is almost universally touted as a wonderful source of protein; in fact, eggs are having a bit of renaissance now. But egg yolks are full of fat and cholesterol. Here's something you can do with your kids: take the yolk out of a hard-cooked egg and rub it between your fingers. Grease. The white of the egg doesn't have the fat and cholesterol, but many times, it has contaminants from chicken feed. A typical egg yolk contains 76 percent fat and 213 milligrams of cholesterol. While fat is an important part of any diet, eggs are not the best source of fat or protein for a variety of reasons. There really is no shortage of fat in the American diet—

and as we discuss throughout this book, there's no shortage of easy, accessible proteins, so no matter what good things can be said about the fat and protein in eggs, we don't need it. Trust us.

The ethical and environmental impact of raising chickens for eggs makes them a tricky business, even in "cage-free" and "cruelty-free" settings. These designations are, in fact, questionable and problematic, as evidenced by the large number of egg recalls, and should not be used as evidence of a "good egg." Bacterial contamination is rampant in the egg industry. Remember when you licked the batter in the bowl as a kid? Those days are done. According to the CDC, *Salmonella* causes more hospitalizations and death than does any other germ found in food and can be found on a perfectly normal-looking egg.[8] In short, just say no to eggs!

Alternatives

There is no egg alternative on the market that replicates a hard-cooked egg, or a fried egg or a sunny-side-up egg, for that matter. However, there are so many egg substitutes that make all kinds of baking possible, tasty, ethically uncomplicated, and super inexpensive. Powdered egg replacers, such as both Ener-G and Bob's Red Mill brand, contain the equivalent of dozens of eggs in one small bag, and all they require is the addition of water to the powder to substitute for eggs in any recipe.

In Chapter 4, we discuss various egg substitutes that you probably already have in your pantry, such as applesauce, mashed banana, and a simple combination of baking powder, oil, and water, which we use all of the time.

Meat-Based Protein

Americans get more than enough protein. The average American male consumes about 100 grams of protein per day, and the average female consumes about 70 grams. Both of these figures are almost twice what the Food and Nutrition Board recommends. For most people, 10 to 15 percent of our daily calories should come from protein, which works out to about 56 grams for men and 46 for women.

Many meat eaters will proudly declare that meat is a superior source of protein. Nutritionally speaking, this is not necessarily so, but it is true that eating a large chunk of any animal meat contains a high concentration of protein. In addition, meat contains many nutrients and minerals, although

Thousands of years ago, nature favored the survival of animals that liked grease. The reason we love the taste of fat is that, over tens of thousands of years, we have acquired a taste for the mouthfeel of it. If you really wanted to survive in prehistoric times, you had to enjoy eating greasy things because you might not get food for another three weeks. If you killed an animal and only ate the lean meat, you wouldn't survive. But if you enjoyed eating woolly mammoth grease, you lived. Of course, cave people only lived to be about twenty-five years old—the oldest Neanderthal appears to have been a little over age thirty. These were the elders—big fat thirty-year-old Neanderthals! They matured very fast, at twice the rate of modern humans.

So it didn't matter how bad grease was. It was good for the first twenty years of your life, and then you were going to die of something else, anyway. Grease and fat are really pretty bad for people who want to live longer than a Neanderthal.

meat is not the only source for these nutrients and minerals.

So what's our beef with meat? We'll look at specific meats in a moment, but here are just a couple of general health concerns about meat.

Go to any government website on food-borne illnesses and disease and see the amount of time devoted to preventing food poisoning from handling raw meat: wash hands with warm soapy water, wash and bleach surfaces, don't cross-contaminate (use separate cutting boards and utensils for meat), cook to a safe temperature, chill promptly, and so on and so forth. You're no more likely to change your baby's poopy diaper on the kitchen counter than we are. But raw meat, they're telling you, on your kitchen counter may be just as dangerous and for similar reasons.

So, cook it, right? Well, one of the main problems with meat is that when you heat it, you create very unnatural chemicals, such as polycyclic and heterocyclic amines (PAHs and HCAs). PAHs come from charred foods such as when you barbecue, and HCAs come from cooking meat proteins at high temperatures, such as in a skillet. Studies show these chemicals are carcinogenic—as in, cancer-causing.

Red Meat

The *New York Times* had a cover story excerpting research published in mid-2012 in the *Archives of Internal Medicine*, showing that people in the upper 20 percent of red meat eaters in America have greater incidence of obesity, cardiovascular disease, and cancer. The next quintile, as they called it, has the same increase to a lesser extent, and on down the line. If you are a non-red meat eater, you minimize your chances of again, obesity, cardiovascular disease, and cancer.[9]

Although not as common as it used to be, hot dogs can still be made with "meat by-products" or "variety meats," which include such things as liver, kidneys, and hearts. Even most of the all-beef and kosher ones are loaded with sodium and fat and nitrates. Hot dogs are just the right shape and size to get caught in the trachea. The American Academy of Pediatrics agrees and called for a reshaping of hot dogs, but fell way short when it forgot to call for reshaping the ingredients, while they were at it.

Chicken, Pork and Fish

CHICKEN: Many people think it's healthier to have chicken as their protein source rather than red meat. Well, take a gander: the average chicken leg, even without the skin, is 30 percent fat, and a skinless thigh is 46 percent fat. And unless you're eating a plain piece of boiled, skinless—and, let's face it—flavorless chicken, you can stop pretending you're saving your health. One of every child's "favorite" foods is chicken nuggets. Fast-food chicken nuggets are made with ammonia-soaked pulverized chicken parts, (yum, yum), petroleum derivatives, and anti-foaming agents, which in addition to being known carcinogens are also flammable—as in: can catch fire. As for "natural" chicken nuggets: they tend to be loaded with fat and sodium. In the long run, chicken's not any healthier than red meat. We've just been told it is. As we mentioned earlier, chickens most often live in terribly crowded conditions and as a result, the CDC's most recent report named chicken as causing the largest proportion of food-borne illness deaths.

PORK: The "other white meat," marketed for its high protein and lean fat, can be just that as long as you're not eating bacon and sausage or some of the other truly fatty parts. But like chickens and cows, pigs are most often raised in crowded, filthy conditions, which means disease, drugs, and ethical issues. Pork comes with all of the same safe-handling rules of poultry and beef and, like chicken, and the leanest parts are pretty much devoid of any true flavor. Stick with the Little Piggies on your toes. And while you're at it, how about changing it from "This little piggie had roast beef," to "roast beets"!

FISH. It's true that fish contains very healthy omega-3s and is a potentially a good edible protein (if it's not an ethical concern for you), but the simple fact is that we have contaminated every good body of water there is. Some fish can live to be anywhere from 5 to 150 years old. Imagine running a strainer through the ocean for 5, 40, or 150 years and seeing what you might catch. Fish skin traps a lot of heavy metals and PCBs, chemicals used in electrical and plastic industries and which were banned in the 1970s. Sadly, they're still out there and in our waters and fish.

The US Food and Drug Administration reported finding illegal levels of methyl mercury in one out of five samples of these types of fish during a three-year review. If it's recommended that you eat something only once a month because it's dangerous, doesn't it just make sense to eat it zero times a month? If something is so toxic that you must limit your consumption, why eat it at all? Go online and check out the number of fish advisories. It paints a pretty tragic picture of pollution and agricultural pesticides that have contaminated almost every river, lake, and stream across America.

State and federal governments warn you to stop eating fish—not just left-wing-alfalfa-eating-tie-dye-shirt-granola advocacy groups. Eating farmed fish isn't really a better alternative because those fish can contain dangerous levels of PCBs because of food that they are fed, and they are raised with the same kind of terrible conditions as factory-farmed chickens—crowded conditions, antibiotics, and chemicals to make them grow faster and fatten them up.

Alternatives

There are two primary sources of protein: animals and plants. There are nine essential amino acids in meat protein, and it used to be thought that the only way to get complete protein from plant-based sources was by eating combinations of vegetables and grains (for instance, rice and beans eaten together, whole wheat bread with hummus, or even rice cakes with a spoonful of almond butter). But reputable nutritionists and medical doctors have long since acknowledged that food combining isn't necessary. Veggies and fruits contain protein—and all forms of protein contain protein-forming amino acids in some quantity. So, basically, if you eat well, you're bound to get all the calories and complete proteins that you need. Your body figures it out. We're not so fragile.

In addition, Americans do not need as much protein as we are told we do by media and campaign ads. If you like statistics and charts, check out the CDC's recommendations at www.cdc.gov/nutrition/everyone/basics/protein.html.

Plant sources of protein include legumes and grains. Protein is found in grains, cereals, pastas, tofu, and beans. Soybeans, from which tofu is made, and quinoa are great sources of protein. Plant-based proteins are easy to make, accessible to all, nutritionally complete, and completely delicious. You can feed your children and yourself with so many other healthy proteins than animal-based ones. For example, beans and nuts are just two sources of proteins that are versatile, easy to use, and

delicious. Non-soy-based veggie burgers are gaining popularity and we have included a few recipes for veggie-style burgers that really satisfy finicky and skeptical appetites.

There are so many tasty and exciting meat alternatives, such as soy-based veggie dogs and veggie burgers, vegan versions of bacon and salami, and just about every "meat" you can imagine. These alternatives are great "transition" foods if you're just exploring a more plant-based diet, and they're super convenient. However, they're also highly processed, so we don't rely on them on a daily basis but eat them sparingly.

Many new vegans are unfamiliar with tempeh and seitan; prepackaged tempeh and seitan are fun and colorful additions to stir-fries, salads, and sandwiches, and they should be tasted in any restaurant you can find that features them on the menu!

Processed Meats

The most recent report by the World Cancer Research Fund (WCRF) confirmed that adults and children who consume processed meats, such as luncheon meats, hot dogs, bacon, and salami, are at a higher risk for cancer. According to the WCRF and the American Institute for Cancer Research

(AICR), the risk of colorectal cancer increases, on average, by 21 percent for every 50 grams (1.7 ounces; think of the size of one typical hot dog) of processed meat consumed daily. The connection between these kinds of meats and cancer was found to be so strong they concluded no amount of processed meats could be considered safe.[10]

According to the National Hot Dog and Sausage Council, on the Fourth of July, Americans will consume (well, they say "enjoy") 150 million hot dogs, enough to stretch from Washington, DC, to L.A. over five times. That's a lot of hot dogs.

Building Up the Vegan Plate (Palate)!

You can get all of the minerals, vitamins, nutrients, and fiber you need from the following plant-based food groups: fruits, vegetables, grains, and legumes. That's it!

Michael Pollan said it best: "Eat food. Not too much. Mostly plant." He just stopped a little short when he said "mostly."

Legumes, which include all the dried beans, such as chickpeas (garbanzos), lentils, lima beans, split peas, kidney beans, and so on, are an excellent source of protein. All the fresh vegetables and fruits give you vitamins and minerals. Grains, such as brown rice, millet, buckwheat, and amaranth, provide protein and fiber. With the exception of vitamin B_{12}, which some vegans take as a supplement once a week (but many don't and are not deficient in, either!), feeding your family from these food groups helps you all to be fit, active and energetic as you're supposed to be, because you won't be filling up on fats. You will have energy that comes from carbohy-

> **DR. JAY:** Everybody complicates nutrition. Nutrition is simple: eat sensible foods. Avoid lots of ingredients. Avoid greasy foods. The ingredients in this apple would be *apple*! Don't get deep-fried apple chips. Don't get things that are made out of processed corn; eat a cob of corn, naturally sweet without anything added. Kids who eat poorly tend to get fat— their fitness suffers, they lose interest in athletics. School gets harder and as they get older; they get teased.[11] They have less fun. Get whole foods to eat. Stop teaching our children to love sugar. And let's try to stop loving sugar ourselves.

drates and natural fruit sugars instead of the truly undesirable hyperactivity that can be triggered by processed sugar.

There is so much research supporting alternative food guidelines, and thankfully, we all get to learn and decide what works for our family nutritionally and also what works for our family's' lifestyle. We provide resources at the back of this book that detail which fruits and vegetables are best for which vitamin, mineral, and nutritional equivalent. Eating a plant-based diet is possible and healthy, and it's also interesting and fun.

You don't need strict guidelines, just use common sense—look at this diagram:

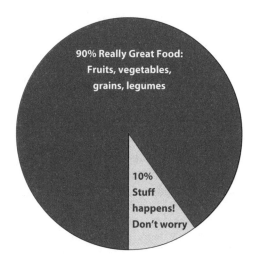

What we really want to do is get everyone to relax, to have fun. By the time this book comes out, someone will have decided that you need more vitamin D or less protein. What we care about is that the plate is attractive to the palate and that what you offer is healthy and enjoyable for your kids and your family. That's why we offer the recipes you'll find in this book. Offer the good stuff and enjoy doing it.

You're the One Who Decides

Food should not be painful to negotiate with your children, and it should not be used as punishment or as the source of struggle. If changes in diet are done gradually and compassionately, kids will adjust. If they seem to not be able to accept even small shifts in food changes and diet, seek the assistance of your pediatrician, licensed nutritionist, or behavioral therapist. It's worth getting the help, and probably you'll benefit as much as they will.

Far too often we've been convinced and sold on feeding our kids terribly. We hear so many parents saying they can "only" feed their kids french fries and chicken fingers or that they "have to" give their kids pizza or fast food. Here's our advice: Take back your role as parent. You're responsible for your family, not advertisers. Not charts made by the government. You get to

COMPARING INGREDIENTS IN AN APPLE WITH LUNCHABLES

As we mentioned before, one of the great things about making your own food is that you know just what is going into your body and your kids. When you don't, it's time to read labels. The more ingredients there are, and the harder the ingredient names get to pronounce, the more serious the crime against real food being committed. Let's compare an apple (which needs no label) to Oscar Mayer's Turkey and Cheddar Sub Lunchable. Go on, we double dare you to read the whole thing.

Apple

Ingredients: Apple

Oscar Mayer—Lunchables—Mega Pack Cracker Combo—Turkey & Cheddar

Servings: 1			
Calories	750	Sodium	1,630 mg
Total Fat	31 g	Potassium	0 mg
Saturated	10 g	Total Carbs	101 g
Polyunsaturated	0 g	Dietary Fiber	2 g
Monounsaturated	0 g	Sugars	57 g
Trans	0 g	Protein	18 g
Cholesterol	40 mg		

	% Daily Value*		% Daily Value*
Vitamin A	6%	Calcium	20%
Vitamin C	4%	Iron	15%

*Percent Daily Values are based on a 2000 calorie diet. Your daily values may be higher or lower depending on your calorie needs.

Ingredients: Water—spring water. Applesauce—apples, apple juice concentrate, water, ascorbic acid (vitamin c). Sub bun—enriched bleached wheat flour ([wheat flour, niacin, reduced iron, thiamin mononitrate , riboflavin , folic acid], malted barley flour), water, sugar, white wheat bran, contains 2% or less of the following: soybean oil, yeast, wheat germ, dough conditioners (mono & diglycerides, sodium stearoyl lactylate, enzyme modified soy lecithin, datem), salt, guar gum, modified cellulose, calcium propionate (preservative), xanthan gum, artificial flavors, enzymes. Contains: wheat, soy. Oven roasted turkey breast—cured-smoked flavor added—browned with caramel color—turkey breast, water, potassium lactate, modified corn starch, contains less than 2% of salt, dextrose, carrageenan, sodium phosphated, sodium diacetate, sodium ascorbate, sodiium nitrite, natural and artificial flavor, smoke flavor, caramel color. 2% milk reduced fat cheddar pasteurized prepared cheese product—pasteurized part-skim milk, water, milkfat, sodium citrate, contains less than 2% of milk protein concentrate, whey protein concentrate, lactic acid, sorbic acid as a preservative, salt, oleoresin paprika (color), annatto (color), vitamin A palmitate, enzymes, cheese culture with starch added for slice separation. Contains: milk. Nilla wafers—unbleached enriched flour (wheat flour, niacin, reduced iron, thiamine mononitrate [vitamin B1], riboflavin [vitamin B2], folic acid), sugar, soybean oil, high fructose corn syrup, partially hydrogenated cottonseed oil, whey (from milk), eggs, natural and artificial flavor, salt, leavening (baking soda and/or calcium phosphate), mono- and diglycerides (emulsifier). Contains: wheat, milk. Egg. Nonfat mayonnaise dressing—water, modified food starch, sugar, high fructose corn syrup, vinegar, soybean oil*, contains less than 2% of salt, cellulose gel, natural flavor, artificial color, egg yolks*, xanthan gum, mustard flour, lactic acid, cellulose gum, phosphoric acid, vitamin E acetate, lemon juice concentrate, dried garlic, dried onions, spice, yellow 6, beta carotene, blue 1, with potassium sorbate and calcium disodium edta as preservatives. Contains: egg. *Trivial source of fat and cholesterol. Tropical punch artificial flavor soft drink mix—sugar, fructose, citric acid (provides tartness), contains less than 2% of natural and artificial flavor, ascorbic acid (vitamin C), vitamin E acetate, calcium phosphate (prevents caking), acesulfame potassium and sucralose (sweeteners), artificial color, red 40, blue 1, BHA (preserves freshness).

When there are this many ingredients you are no longer eating "real food," you are eating substances made to taste like food. Remember Willie Wonka's gum that was a three-course roast beef dinner? It's a brave new world. At least that gum probably didn't have 32 grams of sugar and a whopping 590 milligrams of sodium. Yowza.

decide what you want to do and how you want to eat. There are so many excellent and free resources for you to use to design an eating plan and life that fits your needs, your lifestyle, and your budget. Eating more fruits, vegetables, and grains is something we should all be doing. Limiting salt, sugar, and animal protein is recommended by just about every health organization you can look up. The time is now to learn more, explore more, and find fun ways to create the healthiest and yummiest and easiest ways to eat and feed your family. It's easier than you think.

Notes

1. http://wwwnc.cdc.gov/eid/article/19/3/11-1866_article.htm.

GREAT—*YOU* TRY TO GET MY KID TO NOT WANT FAST FOOD

Dr. Jay does nutritional consultations in his office almost every day, and can attest that families are still taking their children to McDonald's, Burger King, or Kentucky Fried Chicken, even though we all know that fast foods cause obesity and increase a child's (and our own) risk of developing heart disease. The cheap prices and convenience are a cruel temptation for bleary-eyed and overwhelmed parents, though, and once your kids get a taste of it, they'll be clamoring for more (even just the smell is enough to undo ten years of excellent parenting nutrition!). We strongly suggest you eliminate or limit fast food as much as possible. Be strong! It's time to pull out all of the stops here.

2. http://opinionator.blogs.nytimes.com/2012/07/07/got-milk-you-dont-need-it/?_r=0.

3. World Cancer Research Fund/American Institute for Cancer Research, *Food, Nutrition, and the Prevention of Cancer: A Global Perspective* (Washington, DC: American Institute for Cancer Research, 1997), 322; J. M. Chan, M. J. Stampfer, J. Ma, et al., "Dairy Products, Calcium, and Prostate Cancer Risk in the Physicians' Health Study," Presentation, American Association for Cancer Research, San Francisco, April 2000.

4. R. P. Heaney, D. A. McCarron, B. Dawson-Hughes, et al., "Dietary Changes Favorably Affect Bone Remodeling in Older Adults," *Journal of the American Dietary Association* 99 (1999): 1228–33.

5. The milk industry's newer target group is teens, with its "Body By Milk" campaign spotlighting teen sports and entertainment stars.

6. http://www.nlm.nih.gov/medlineplus/ency/article/007134.htm; P. Cohen, " Serum Insulin-like Growth Factor-I levels and Prostate Cancer Risk—Interpreting the Evidence," *Journal of the National Cancer Institute* 90 (1998): 876–79; J. Cadogan, R. Eastell, N. Jones, and M. E. Barker, "Milk Intake and Bone Mineral Acquisition in Adolescent Girls: Randomised, Controlled Intervention Trial," *BMJ* 315 (1997): 1255–60.

7. http://www.vrg.org/nutrition/calcium.php.

8. http://www.cdc.gov/features/salmonellaineggs.

9. http://www.nytimes.com/2012/03/13/health/research/red-meat-linked-to-cancer-and-heart-disease.html.

10. http://www.dietandcancerreport.org.

11. J. Lumeng et al., "Weight Status as a Predictor of Being Bullied in Third Through Sixth Grades" *Pediatrics* 2010; DOI: 10.1542/peds.2009-0774, http://pediatrics.aappublications.org/cgi/content/abstract/peds.2009-0774v1.

DR. JAY: Just say no to "have to's" with food:

- You don't have to make it all gone.

- You don't have to eat it if you don't want to.

- You don't have to finish it to get dessert.

- You don't have to like an assortment of vegetables (the doctor who coauthored this book didn't like any of them until he was twenty-two years old).

- You don't have to eat one item to get to eat another.

- You don't have to do something to get food as a reward.

- You don't have to have done something "bad" to get food as a punishment.

- You don't have to be sad or disappointed to get something sweet and yummy to eat.

- You don't have to finish your lunch to grow (let them eat their lunch on the car ride home when food is competing with playtime).

- You don't have to eat three meals a day. Sometimes you'll prefer to eat many small meals over the course of the day.

- You don't have to become a healthy eater overnight. A slow but steady evolution is just fine with us.

- And you don't have to have an ice cream just because you hear the jingling truck!

CHAPTER 3

What Do We Actually Eat?
Easy Meal Tips

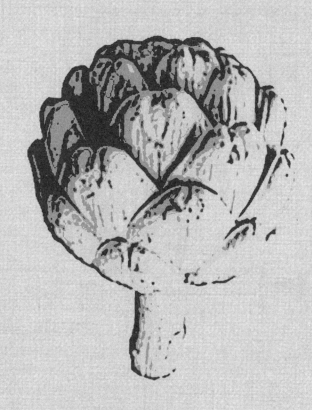

We've established that all the vitamins, minerals, proteins, and fats you need to be nutritionally healthy are obtainable through a plant-based diet, and evidence is continuing to support that not eating meat and dairy is good for your heart, good for your brain, and good for the planet. That being said, there is still a lot of confusion about a vegan diet and we get asked a lot, "What do you actually eat?" This is a great question, and although the answer varies from person to person and family to family, we want to present some of the general guidelines we use for preparing meals and snacks.

The kind of nutrition we advocate for isn't going to be available 100 percent of the time, and we know that. There are birthday parties. (You are probably not going to be the family that brings a bag of carrots to every birthday party. You don't want your child to be nicknamed "Carrot Boy from the Birthday Party.") There are holidays. There are probably going to be a few dozen days a year when your kid eats junky stuff. (Dr. Jay always used to tell friends that if his daughter was going to their kid's birthday party and they were going to give her cookies, cake, ice cream, 7UP, and a piñata full of candy, to keep her overnight because on the car ride home, the kid

was gonna be a mess!) But the other 329-plus days can be easy. Your child can open the refrigerator and be looking at watermelon, and apples, and carrots, all cut up and convenient, for dessert or snacks. You can offer and serve delicious foods that we'll help you to make right here. So, okay. Let's go!

Breakfast

It is said that breakfast is the most important meal of the day, and nutritionally speaking, that's pretty true. After a night of sleeping and reduced metabolic activity, breakfast is the meal that gets blood sugar (energy) into your bloodstream which allows your brain to start firing, your muscles to start working, and your day to start with a bang. Even though most prepackaged "traditional" breakfast products, such as pancakes, waffles, and even a lot of breakfast breads and rolls, contain milk and eggs and a lot of sugar, breakfast is not a difficult meal for vegans. Dr. Jay himself admits that he can't cook, but he used to make pancakes for his daughter from scratch without milk or eggs, using almond milk and blueberries for some pizzazz. A little creativity can go a long way! So can bucking conventional notions of what's appropriate for breakfast—it can lead to a wider set of choices for your plant-based breakfast. For example, there's nothing wrong with bean soup for breakfast, or miso soup and brown rice, or a big, delicious salad. It may take some time to get your kids used to it, but the options are endless. Kids love the idea of unconventional breakfasts, as evidenced by their institutionalized "backward day" at schools. In addition, there's nothing that says that breakfast has to be elaborate and supply all of the day's protein every day every week. But just because we don't eat eggs or bacon or ham, doesn't mean we don't also get protein in our breakfasts. Having an open mind, and remembering that there is protein in oats and granola and even a rice and bean burrito can keep everyone going strong, all morning long.

Here are some of our breakfast guidelines.

1. KEEP IT SIMPLE FOR KIDS. Put some freshly cut fruit with a handful of raw almonds in front of your kids and watch them chow down, especially if you arrange the fruit and nuts attractively or, as Mayim prefers, in awesome shapes, such as her famous "Fruit Face" breakfast that her boys love. Presenting kids with three or four choices of cut fruit is a great way to start their day. Bananas are especially filling, mangoes are a great sweet breakfast treat, berries are a terrific option, too, and if you have a set of fun toothpicks and cool plates, we guarantee the fruit on those plates will disappear pretty quickly into happy tummies.

2. GET SMOOTH. Breakfast is a great opportunity to present fresh fruits and vegetables in the form of smoothies. Smoothies are filling, simple to make, and easy to transport for car rides and walks about. Smoothies can be breakfast for as many days a week as you want them to be! In our families we have three or four smoothie and juice recipes that we know everyone can agree on, and it's always wonderful to watch kids essentially drink a cup of spinach, because you know it's healthy for them and they know that with a banana and some frozen berries, it's just yummy! Smoothies in particular have a ton of fiber and they are a great way to start the day "regular." Juices and smoothies are wonderful carriers for additions of things that certain people find hard to stomach, such as wheatgrass (for fiber and vitamins), lemon and ginger (for a healthy digestive system), or a shot of omega 3–rich supplemental oils (Mayim sneaks flaxseed oil into her boys' smoothies

> **DR. JAY:** Adults can change their palate overnight, if they have to. For children, it can take over a year. You may need to transition these flavors over a week, or five or ten or more. You can't switch taste buds that fast. There's no urgency. Give new flavors and textures time. Kids come back around, but you don't change them with coercion. You change them by leading by example. You change them by making it interesting and keeping it fun and by transitioning slowly.

on most days and no one is the wiser!) They are also a great way to get in extra servings of greens by including milder greens, such as spinach or romaine lettuce, with fruit and nondairy milk. For protein and extra calories, if you want them, nut butters can be added (banana, almond butter, and spinach? Think healthy, rich, delicious shake).

3. COLD CEREAL. If a cereal-like feeling really starts your morning right, think about making your own granola. It's easy to do—the ingredients are simple (oats and nuts with a touch of maple syrup and brown sugar)—and

you can make large batches to store in airtight containers (check out Mayim's favorite GRANOLA recipe on PAGE 62). We try not to do cold cereal more than two mornings a week, because it's high in carbohydrates and lower on vitamins and minerals than, say, a smoothie.

4. HOT CEREAL! Whole oats prepared on the stove top with a little blackstrap molasses (a great source of iron and calcium) is another simple, quick, and inexpensive way to start the day, especially on chilly mornings. Additions of nuts and raisins enhance the taste and visual appeal, and small hands love "dressing up" their breakfast this way. Older kids will love the taste and energy it gives them.

And there's nothing wrong with a little bit of maple syrup and blueberries—but the person in charge of the maple syrup has to have a driver's license or be over eighteen. It's meant to be sprinkled on, not glug-glugged.

And although the "instant" packets may be tempting, most contain preservatives and a lot of sugar. It's great to get kids (and adults, too!) used to the pure taste of simple foods. You can always transition from using processed sugary oatmeal to one-half packaged and one-half whole oats, and then gradually decrease (over the course of a week or two, for example) to whole

SHOW AND TELL: STARTING YOUR DAY RIGHT

Here's how Dr. Jay explains it to kids: I show kids with my hand what their "blood energy" looks like when they're sleeping—low, *you're sleeping!*—and what happens when they start their day with a big strawberry doughnut or sugar-frosted cocoa blech cereal: a mountainlike steep rise and a fast drop to below zero. So in an hour, their body will need another strawberry jelly doughnut. And then I ask them whether they really want to try to play soccer, dance, or walk through school with a pocket filled with those sugary strawberry doughnuts.

When they realize that sticky pockets aren't the best way to get through the day, I tell them how a balance of protein, such as a handful of nuts or a protein shake with some fruit, gives a nice quick energy rise (I raise my hand) and then levels off until (I dip my hand) it's time for a snack and then lunch. This little show gives them the idea that eating sugar might give them a minute of crazy energy but it's gone quickly and fun lasts too long to be fueled by sugary junk.

With older kids, it's pretty easy to explain that sugar doesn't give their body what it needs for sports. I think I can find something in all kids' lives that will motivate them to want to be more skilled (faster, stronger, faster again) than they are right now. I tell them, "You don't get there with cookies, cakes, candy and sugar-frosted cocoa blech. Eat like the athlete you want to be!"

oats with naturally sweet additions. Plain whole oats contain less sugar than granolas, so this is a safe bet for a few mornings a week.

5. STARCHY TREATS. We try to discourage excessively starchy and sugary breakfasts, and instead make it a priority to incorporate good solid protein

in the morning hours. See Dr. Jay's box "Show and Tell: Starting Your Day Right" on page 35 for why sugary treats in the morning just don't pan out.

Breakfast breads, such as banana bread or muffins or bagels, can be frozen and reheated as needed; if you're going this route in the morning, try to work toward also incorporating protein-rich foods, such as nuts, nut butters, and tofu, into breakfasts.

Of course, pancakes are fun on some mornings, and since they generally are not vegan-friendly at most stores or restaurants, many families will whip up their own dry pancake mix in larger amounts and store it in an airtight container. Mayim has "Pancake Fridays" for her boys, and all she has to do is add a little oil, some nondairy milk or water, and one egg's worth of egg replacer, and pancakes are ready for the table in minutes.

Lunch

In general, lunch should be protein and energy-rich, but not too time consuming to prepare. Lunches for kids often need to fit into a lunchbox; weekend or "lazy day" lunches can be more elaborate. We like to follow the more European style of a larger and more substantial lunch on weekends, with a lighter dinner. This tends to allow us to burn off the calories of a large meal throughout the afternoon and into the evening, whereas eating a large dinner leaves us with a belly full of food just in time to get ready to settle down for the night, which can set us up for indigestion, acid reflux, and other such lovely side effects of lying down with too much food in our tummy! In addition, the cleanup from a large dinner often becomes a struggle when bedtime approaches, whereas cleaning up after a large lunch is more likely to recruit the help of the others in the family. Lunch is a great opportunity to try new things, such as browsing a market's produce aisle for new ideas or seeing what kind of prepared vegan foods strike your fancy. Although processed vegan products such as veggie bacon, salami, and hot dogs should not be consumed in excess, you might find that you like them once in a while and they may be a good standby for meals in a pinch. Mayim, despite her initial reluctance, recently made a delicious "mock tuna fish" with mashed chickpeas, vegan mayonnaise, and some delicately diced dill pickles; even seasoned vegans sometimes need to step outside of their comfort zone! (Speaking of mock tuna, here's Dr. Jay's favorite "tuna" sandwich: Mix 3 to 4 tablespoons of

Worried about whether your kids aren't eating lunch at school? Kids eat when they're hungry—and they'll eat the good stuff you give them.

Dr. Jay asked a five-year-old and a ten-year-old similar questions. Five: "When the bell rings at lunchtime, would you rather eat lunch or go out and play?" He looked at Dr. Jay as if he was crazy: "Play!"

The ten-year-old is a serious hoopster; Dr. Jay asked whether he'd rather eat lunch or play ball. He responded politely but pretty certainly: "Not enough for five on five? Play half court. No game? Hang out and talk with friends." His choice number twelve? Eat lunch.

Or take a page from Dr. Jay's wife, Meyera, a chef: when their daughter Simone was about twelve years old, someone asked Meyera what she made Simone for her school lunches. Simple: "Whatever I'd like her to eat on the ride home when I pick her up at four o'clock."

hummus with chopped celery and tomatoes. Spread on two slices of preferably gluten-free bread. Enjoy!)

Here are some of our favorite lunch ideas:

1. EMBRACE SIMPLICITY. Although it's great to punctuate our weeks with a few special and elaborate dishes, many of the recipes in this book are not things we make every single day. By and large, vegan eating (and lunches in particular) can and should be very simple. Especially when feeding small mouths, try to have lunch contain a hearty protein, a vegetable or fruit component, and a healthy carbohydrate. One of our favorite lunches for small and big appetites alike is a fantastic burrito. A tortilla (whole wheat or sprouted grain is our preference), beans (from the can or soaked and cooked if you are feeling adventurous), sliced-up veggies (raw or sautéed in a little garlic or olive oil), and a little pizzazz (a sprinkle of vegan cheese, sour cream, or salsa, for example), and you are done. As an

aside, we are generally not advocates of making "different" meals for everyone in the house. Our general plan of attack is to present a few choices at each meal, with options for creativity and individualizing the meal. In Mayim's house, whoever doesn't like what's on the table can ask for anything raw in the house, such as any vegetable or fruit or nuts. It works!

2. SALAD CENTERPIECE. Dr. Jay has taught Mayim's kids—and countless other kids as well—to eat a salad "as big as your head" every day. Mayim's boys get so excited when they do just that because they know Dr. Jay will be thrilled. (They also think it's awesome that their heads are smaller than Dr. Jay's and he has to eat a much bigger salad than they do!) Basing a lunch around a hearty salad presents great opportunities for many appetites to be satisfied. We like to present a bunch of options for salad toppings, such as various diced veggies, nuts, croutons, or canned beans and corn (for a Mexican TACO SALAD, for example, see PAGE 87), so that everyone's salad can be customized. It's great to have a few tasty vegan salad dressings on hand for people to choose from, or better yet, make your own from any combination of the following ingredients: olive oil, balsamic vinegar, mustard, agave nec-

tar, garlic, and freshly squeezed lemon juice. Alongside a salad centerpiece, we sometimes have MINESTRONE SOUP (PAGE 79); CHILI (PAGE 152); a hearty bread, such as corn bread (we present a few great versions of CORN BREAD on PAGE 166); or even a smaller plate, such as a fried vegetable and potato LATKE (PAGE 129), which might be too heavy and rich to serve on its own as a main course but can be delightful when presented with a healthy and filling salad as the main event (such as greens and croutons with a choice of DRESSINGS, PAGES 82, 84, 86, 92, 94, 95).

3. LAZY DAYS. On lazy days at home or weekends, we love to have a pot of chili or some sort of veggie stew on the stove (see VEGGIE CHILI on PAGE 152). Once you figure out your family's preferences, stews can be a great standby that are also able to be prepared in large batches and frozen, or made with minimal effort in a slow cooker. Chilis are especially popular with vegans because of the high protein content in beans, and they are also a wonderful way to sneak in a ton of vegetables while making small people happy with all of the condiments they get to use, dressing up their chili bowl however they like it by adding onions, a drop of vegan cheese or sour cream, avocado chunks, or salsa.

4. **Box it up.** One of Mayim's closest friends and earliest advocates for vegan living (she also is the photographer for this book!) used to send her boys to Mayim's house with the most hilarious lunches, or so it seemed to Mayim at the time. The lunchboxes contained such things as a bushel of tangerines, a bag of almonds, and enough raw carrots, cucumbers, and celery to feed a village of happy rabbits. Mayim marveled at how content these kids were to eat all this amazing healthy and simple food, and now she looks to those lunchboxes as a model for ideal easy meals for her boys. Now, it's true that not all kids will enjoy that kind of lunchbox, but more conventional lunchbox plans can follow the model of nonvegan lunchboxes to a certain extent. Kids love sandwiches, and we tend to go for lower-fat, higher-protein spreads, such as almond butter or sunflower butter, on a nice hearty whole wheat bread. Instead of prepackaged processed snacks, such as chips or gummy animal-shaped things, vegan lunchboxes can contain all the yummy foods we have been talking about teaching kids to love early: almonds, carrots and hummus, apple slices, and any other fruit that can be neatly and easily packaged. Fun foods can be pretzels, roasted nuts, or carefully selected but healthy sweets, such as the awesome and tasty RAISIN APRICOT SUPER ENERGY BARS you'll find on PAGE 66.

Food should not be used as punishment, nor should eating times be stressful and full of strife. If you are having a lot of food struggles with your kids, we recommend speaking to your pediatrician, a licensed nutritionist, or a family therapist. Often, other issues are at play if you are struggling with your kids over food, and a licensed professional can help you sort them out.

What we don't recommend is this approach: "Take two bites of this food you dislike and we'll reward you with food that will be an unhealthy habit for the rest of your life."

5. **Fun food day.** In Mayim's family, Saturday is the Jewish Sabbath and this is the day when lunch becomes a feast of sorts. For many families, weekends are an opportunity to have a special big lunch, and this doesn't have to mean a lot of work or stress. Mayim tends to make Saturday a "fun food" day, by serving dishes that require a little more effort or tend to be a little more calorie-rich. Examples include VEGAN FRENCH ONION DIP (made with vegan sour cream and mayonnaise and dried onions, dill, and garlic, PAGE 116); a heavier dish, such as vegan MAC N CHEEZ casserole (PAGE 132); or CHALLAH (traditional braided bread, PAGE 174). Many vegan families don't make dessert an everyday event, but selecting one day a week when there is a dessert option makes dessert a special and selective event, rather than an expected or too frequent one that can lead to sugar meltdowns all week long! Others feel that offering dessert in moderation keeps it from becoming a "forbidden fruit" that becomes the center of the show. And speaking of fruit, a lot of the time, kids' thresholds can be set to love natural sweet stuff for dessert. We can show kids that there's *real* sweet, such as an excellent apple, great berries or watermelon, as compared with a *fake* sweet, such as commercially sold sweetened raspberry puree or processed sugary cookies. Raspberries all on their own taste incredibly sweet unless you eat Oreos an hour earlier.

Dinner

The iconic images of families sitting down together every night for a big happy calm dinner are for many families a thing of the past, and dinnertime can often be a stressful time of the day, at least in our experience. There is homework to be done, baths to take, a spouse to reconnect with, and general winding down. Sitting down for a meal together is often the hardest thing to have happen! It would be disingenuous for us to say that dinner is not important and that you don't need to share it as a family. As much as possible, dinner is a great time to reconnect as a family. However, even if that happens only one or two nights a week, that's great, too.

The guidelines for dinner don't have to be significantly different from those we have offered for lunch. Here are a few extra tips for dinners.

1. **One-bowl happiness.** One of the best ways to let kids (and adults) feel a

positive sense of control and a healthy relationship with their food is to do one-bowl meals where customizing is up to each eater. TACO SALAD (PAGE 87) is a great example of presenting a bunch of options for a salad along with condiments and a variety of flavors and colors to choose from. Another great example is a SUSHI IN A BOWL (PAGE 146) that can also be customized according to personal tastes. Even our recipe for BANH MI (PAGE 98), although not a one-bowl meal, can be presented with a variety of great toppings that offer everyone a choice. When a bunch of healthy toppings and options are available and there are a few fun dressings and sauces to choose from, everyone wins.

2. CONTAINMENT. Although sandwiches are thought of mostly as a lunchtime meal, they can actually be a really smart choice for dinner. Why? Well, they tend to have a few basic ingredients: the outside (bun, tortilla, bread), the inside (whatever your "meat" is), and the bells and whistles (condiments, dressings). This means all you really have to prepare is the "meat" of the meal, and then you slap it inside its outside and let everyone select the bells and whistles according to taste. We have some great recipes in

this very book for substantial and delicious, dinner-appropriate sandwiches, such as a killer VEGAN REUBEN (PAGE 102), QUINOA BURGERS (PAGE 97), and healthy CHICKPEA BURGERS (PAGE 100), which we have known small children to eat three of in a sitting. Containing dinner this way helps contain chaos in the house, we promise.

3. THE POWER OF FUN. There are foods kids—and adults—will eat just about anytime. These foods happen to be the ones that almost every nonvegan parent claims they or their kids "can't live without" in the same breath that they say that these foods are "all they will eat!" Well, we know that's not really true, but we also know that the following foods make people very, very happy: pizza, "chicken" fingers (chickens don't have fingers, Dr. Jay likes to point out), and grilled cheese. It's totally fine to have a night or two a week of fun foods that you also pack with nutritional punch when no one's looking. We have some great examples of ways to make PIZZA a much more fulfilling experience nutritionally, while still keeping the fun (check out PAGES 149–150). Although we tend to shy away from processed vegan "chicken" fingers, there are some nights when we serve them, as long as there is broccoli

or a baked parsnip "fry" served with them. Same goes for grilled cheese, made with store-bought vegan cheese; moreover, there are ways to increase the nutritional quality of a grilled cheese sandwich. One of Mayim's favorite things to do is to load up grilled cheese with spinach, kale, or sunflower sprouts and watch how even a little bit of shredded vegan cheese makes all of those fun greens super palatable!

4. LEFTOVERS! As we've mentioned, there is nothing wrong with serving simple meals at any time of day. Dinnertime can be made much less stressful if you reimagine lunch from earlier in the day, or from a previous day! We have been known to add a new set of burrito filling options for dinner, or dice up some spinach and put all of the lunchtime burrito fillings onto the spinach as "taco salad" dinner. Soups or chilis served with a "new" (i.e., the only thing you made new for the meal) side dish are just as good for dinner as they were for lunch. Remember your friend and ours, the slow cooker? It makes enough for dinner and some leftovers, so embrace the slow cooker! Leftovers are your friends. Use them, and use this also as an opportunity to gently remind your kids that the home

is not the same as a restaurant and we all get to be grateful to be a part of the family meal, even if it involves leftovers!

Snacks

A lot of people worry that they'll be hungry all the time if they go vegan. While we understand the theoretical concern, as vegans who love snacking, we have found things that always keep us satisfied and energized. Snacks don't have to be elaborate; in fact, they shouldn't be. Dr. Jay relies on almonds, apples, dried apricots, pretzels, and occasional soy chips, healthy energy bars, popcorn, and almond milk smoothies with vegan protein powder to keep him going through his workday. Some of our favorite snacks are rice cakes with nut butter, raw fruits and veggies, and anything you can dip or eat on the run. Trying to avoid a lot of processed foods means we have to get a little creative to find things that are good in a pinch, but with some good preplanning, snacktime can be super fun and successful for vegan families—kids and adults alike.

1. GO RAW. Fruits and vegetables are awesome snacks at any time of the day.

It's so important to get yourself and your palate used to the taste and texture of simple raw foods. The most commonly reached-for fruits are apples and pears and bananas and berries and grapes, but a whole world of fruits is waiting for you to explore and enjoy, fruits that are even more exciting and contain even more nutrients than you thought possible from a fruit. Unusual examples we have grown to love are mangoes, kiwis, and lychees (yes, the slimy things that come in that awesome scarlet-colored spiky seed pod). Carrots and celery are a great snack, especially when paired with a protein-rich dip, such as hummus, nut butter, or a nutty vegan cheese, but cucumbers, zucchini, and bell peppers also love to be dipped, too, so make it happen!

Cardboard isn't raw and juice boxes don't count as a fruit. Juice boxes are full of sugar. Any vitamins and minerals that you once found in that apple juice have long been forsaken for the sugars. Excessive juice consumption can cause cavities, diarrhea, and bloating, and the American Pediatric Association suggests that "intake of fruit juice should be limited to 4 to 6 oz/day for children 1 to 6 years old, and to 8 to 12 oz or 2 servings per day for children 7 to 18 years old."[1] The biggest problem—we've bet you've already noticed—is that once you give your kids juice boxes, it's very hard to convince them to drink water instead. In fact, bring a pack of preschoolers to a picnic and have juice boxes on the menu and sometimes that's all they'll "eat." Freshly squeezed juices diluted with water are better. When these are served immediately after juicing, many of the vitamins and minerals remain. Still, better than any juice is a piece of fresh fruit with all of the sweetness and added benefit of the fibers.

2. Go nuts. Vegans need protein. We also need fat, but not too much. Raw nuts are a great way to get protein, minerals, nutrients, and just the right amount of fat. Making your own trail mix and storing it in a container in your pantry is a great place to start: combine a few handfuls each of walnuts, almonds, cashews, sunflower seeds, raisins—you can experiment with different combos, including dried fruits (apple chips, banana, coconut), and dates for a sweet touch. A handful or so of nuts at a time is a good rule of thumb for a snack, and when combined with fruit, it makes for a really smart and complete snack that is delicious and filling. Apple slices and walnuts, tangerines and almonds—you get

the picture. As we will show in some of our recipes, soaking nuts in water for a few hours and blending them in a processor with some basic spices turns nuts into spreadable pâtélike deliciousness, as in the RAW NUT CHEESE (PAGE 111). Nuts are your new best friend!

3. GO EASY. Put a dollop of nut butter in the middle of an apple and bake it in the oven for a well-balanced and super easy snack. Air-popped popcorn has to be one of the last great simple pleasures in this world, and although it's fun to drizzle some vegan margarine over popcorn sometimes, it's also great to serve some regular air-popped popcorn as a fun snack, or especially for kids' parties. You can toy with different flavor combos—maple syrup and a touch of sea salt for a caramel or kettle corn taste, nutritional yeast and olive oil for a cheesier taste, or even a splash of soy sauce.

These are just some examples for quick and easy foods; as you experiment more in your kitchen, you'll find out what foods are best for your family, schedule, and budget. Cook the good food that you know is going to be healthy for your family for a long time to come, and wait for them to keep on trying it. At times it will be tricky. At times it won't be perfect. Just relax and have fun! Your kids will find all the right foods if you keep on offering it to them, and in the process so will you. As we've been saying all along, there are so many great plant-based food options, you may have trouble trying them all!

> **DR. JAY:** A note about kids and nuts: kids and nuts don't mix for the first years, but you can start adding ground nuts to certain foods as desired, after the age of one year. At age one, kids can eat everything in the family's diet except two groups of food: unhealthy food we wish we had never learned to like as kids (think french fries, potato chips, and candy), and small hard foods (such as nuts and seeds), which fit right up a child's nostril (yes, they do) and can also end up in the trachea. Once they are old enough to manage chewing and grinding, walnuts are great (as they tend to be the softest), as are pistachios and pumpkin seeds—at around three years of age.

Notes

1. Committee on Nutrition: "The Use and Misuse of Fruit Juice in Pediatrics," AAP Policy: *Journal of the American Academy of Pediatrics* 107, no. 5: 1210. Accessed November 2, 2010. http://aappolicy.aap publications.org/cgi/content/full/pediatrics ;107/5/1210#Recommendation.

CHAPTER 4

What's in Our Kitchens and Cupboards? Stocking a Plant-Based Kitchen

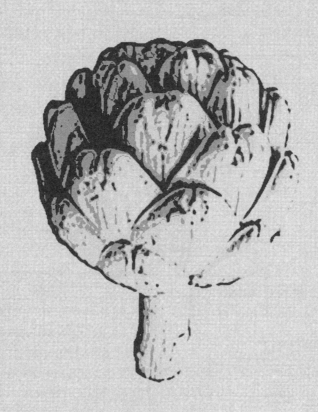

Making a transition to a plant-based diet doesn't just affect what you eat and where you eat, it also affects how you shop and how you stock your refrigerator, freezer, and pantry. The general goals of a vegan kitchen and pantry are to use organic when possible, avoid products with ingredients you can't pronounce, and use the "rule of thumb": if the ingredients list is longer than your thumb (held horizontal for the purist and vertical for the novice), don't buy it. In addition, if you don't have salty, sugary, junky stuff in your house, you won't have to fight with your kids—or yourself!—about it. For those with kids who are very used to having that stuff on hand, a solid week of their asking for it and your gently reminding them that it's not in the house will do the trick and we can guarantee, they will stop asking and move on.

If you're new to plant-based eating, you might think you have to go out and buy a bunch of overpriced ingredients. We keep it simple: while there are some ingredients that might be new to you, all of them are easy to find. The lists begin with some of our favorite fruits and veggies (especially ones we use in our recipes) and move on to basic kitchen staples that will make preparing great vegan food easy, fun, and economical.

Fruit

APPLES, PEARS, GRAPES, PLUMS, PLUOTS, PEACHES, APRICOTS, MELONS: Nature's packaged snacks! We always try to keep seasonal fresh fruit on hand.

STRAWBERRIES, BLUEBERRIES, RASPBERRIES: Fresh berries are great for snacking on, as well as for adding to breakfasts or as a natural dessert. Frozen berries are especially handy for making smoothies colorful, sweet, and full of nutritional goodness. (Note that berry allergies should be discussed with your pediatrician before introducing any berries to babies or small children.)

BANANAS: One of the most versatile fruits around. They can be used in vegan baking and in smoothies to heighten consistency and provide a great source of vitamins, too. They're great to have on hand in the freezer for instant smoothie bliss.

AVOCADOS: This vegan staple is full of healthy fats, protein, and vitamins. Avocados can and ought to be enjoyed au naturel, simply sliced on toast or greens, but they also become everyone's favorite dip when you combine them with some onion, garlic, lime juice, and cilantro (guacamole anyone?). Avocado season is our favorite time of year, hands down.

CUCUMBER: Feels like a vegetable, but is actually a fruit. Regardless of what it is, it's another great snack food, especially if cut into rounds and dipped into hummus.

LEMON: Great for last-minute seasoning and making dressings and sauces.

TOMATOES: Raw, cooked, baked, turned into sauce—you name it, a tomato can be it.

Dried Fruits

RAISINS, PRUNES, APRICOTS, DATES: Perfect for a natural sweet snack, as well as for use in trail mix, granola, and iron-rich recipes, such the ENERGY BARS on PAGE 66.

Vegetables

CARROTS, CELERY: Terrific raw as a snack, or for dipping into hummus, nut butter, or vegan cheese.

CORN: Fresh works well for salads or grilling; frozen is wonderful to have on hand, too, for salads, or just defrosted as an easy side dish.

ONIONS, GARLIC: These are the key ingredients for creating new flavors and starting off any recipe right by sautéing both in 2 tablespoons of olive oil.

BROCCOLI: Wonderful raw or steamed. Also great in stir-fries, or added to salads for some extra nutritional punch.

BELL PEPPER: Another versatile veg that's delicious raw or cooked—for salads, stir-fries, or dipping into spreads, such as hummus.

SCALLION: Adds a little pizzazz to your salads and casseroles.

SQUASH (CROOKNECK, YELLOW, GREEN): Squash can be baked with a little olive oil and some herbs, or cubed for use in quinoa or rice, or sliced and baked like fancy french fries. The possibilities are almost endless! If you want to get really fancy, fried squash blossoms stuffed with vegan cheese make a decadent treat.

CANNED/FROZEN VEGGIES: We love fresh produce but you can't beat organic canned tomatoes for a quick homemade red sauce. Frozen greens are delicious added to smoothies. Just make sure to look for organic and those without added funky flavors

THE DIRTY DOZEN PLUS AND THE CLEAN FIFTEEN

The Environmental Working Group (www.ewg.org/foodnews/summary.php) offers a list of what is known as the Dirty Dozen Plus—that is, the dozen fruits and vegetables most likely to be contaminated with pesticides, along with an additional two crops that are also commonly contaminated. These are the ones to aim for when buying organic, if possible:

Apples	Potatoes
Celery	Spinach
Cherry tomatoes	Strawberries
Cucumbers	Sweet bell peppers
Grapes	
Hot peppers	PLUS:
Nectarines (imported)	Kale/collard greens
Peaches	Summer squash

The Clean Fifteen are the fifteen least contaminated fruits and vegetables that—if you have to pick and choose—are a safer bet to eat from nonorganic sources:

Asparagus	Mangoes
Avocados	Mushrooms
Cabbage	Onions
Cantaloupe	Papayas
Sweet corn	Pineapples
Eggplant	Sweet peas (frozen)
Grapefruit	Sweet potatoes
Kiwi	

(extra salt, I'm looking at you) or preservatives. BPA-free boxed options of veggies are starting to pop up in some supermarkets.

Dairy Substitutes

RICE MILK/ALMOND MILK/SOY MILK: There are many choices for milk substitutes, and which you pick will depend on your taste and your sweet tooth. Almond milk tends to be sweeter and thicker than rice milk, and "original" and vanilla (and even chocolate!) varieties are available in all milk substitutes. We don't generally stock soy milk in our pantry, as a lot of negative attention is being given to processed soy. While some recipes in this book call for processed soy, we prepare them sparingly and don't try to make soy an everyday food. Note that some of the flavored varieties of all of these milks (and even those labeled "plain") tend to contain sugar or another sweetener, but there are plenty of unsweetened options, too.

VEGAN MARGARINE (WE LIKE EARTH BALANCE): A butter substitute is important to have for baking, and it's also great to be able to have the feeling of spreading something butter-like on a bagel or piece of toast once in a while.

We like Earth Balance because it's lower in chemicals than a lot of commercially processed margarines, and it also comes in a soy-free and organic variety now, too.

VEGAN SOUR CREAM: It's not something to use every day, but one dollop in chili or on a taco salad (as a dressing of sorts) makes unhappy children (and skeptical adults!) happy and willing to eat what's in front of them.

Nuts and Seeds, Beans, and Grains,

ALMONDS, WALNUTS AND CASHEWS: Excellent for snacking, in granola, and for making nut butters.

SOY NUTS, PISTACHIOS, AND PEANUTS: Great to have on hand, but not used as regularly as almonds, walnuts, and cashews. These are good for adding to trail mix or for using in specific recipes, but as nuts can go rancid quickly, you may not need to buy these in the same quantities you would the others.

NUT BUTTERS: As with nondairy milks, there are lots of options here, including almond butter, peanut butter, and sunflower butter; having some nut butter available makes for a variety of great quick (and protein-rich) sandwiches and snacks.

WHEAT GERM AND FLAXSEED: These are used for sprinkling over oats, into smoothies, and into pancake batter, breads, and even cookies. Wheat germ is super healthy for your heart and flaxseeds are one of the best sources of omegas for people who don't get omegas from fish and eggs. You can typically buy ground flaxseeds (the best way to get the most nutrients from flaxseeds is to eat them ground) for about the same price as whole, which means you don't have to grind them yourself.

BEANS: We like to have all and any kind of canned beans on hand, and some dried beans as well. Black (plain and refried), kidney, pinto, baked (rinse off most of the sugary fun sauce they typically come in and combine them with a can of rinsed plain pinto beans; no one will be the wiser); beans are perfect on their own, in a salad, as a salad, in a burrito or taco, for breakfast, lunch, or dinner. Beans. We can't get enough of them, and soaking beans and cooking them, while time consuming, does make a world of difference for flavor. Most of the time, though, many of us use canned or boxed beans—and that's okay, too!

QUINOA: Quinoa is your friend. It is the highest-protein grainlike seed in the world, takes the least resources to grow and harvest, can take on the flavor of anything (just like rice), and can be bought in bulk. It's easy to make (just rinse it in a colander, add water that is double the amount of the quinoa you put in, and cook for 20 minutes). It comes in black, red, and that irresistible pale cream color. Quinoa hot, quinoa cold, quinoa subtle, quinoa bold. Make it happen!

ROLLED OATS: Oats aren't just a wonderful breakfast; they can also be the basis for hearty and healthy breads, cookies, and muffins.

RICE: Brown rice is a great source of fiber and protein, and for the stubborn among you, go ahead and have some white rice on hand, too. Just don't let kids get too used to the white variety; it's hard to make them switch back!

PASTA: Pasta is always going to be a great go-to for meals, especially for kids. Whole wheat pasta, like brown rice, is a great source of fiber and protein, but for the occasional treat, go crazy and have white pasta around, too. When Mayim makes her MAC N CHEEZ casserole (PAGE 132), she uses white pasta and loves every blessed bite of it! Gluten-free pastas used to be crumbly and unpredictable, but so many companies now make excellent, firm gluten-free alternatives. They're definitely worth trying out.

Condiments

OIL: Olive oil is a wonderful choice for baking and sautéing, as well as for making dressings and sauces. We also recommend having sesame oil around as a different flavor for dressings and vegetables in particular, and a healthy canola oil as well, for recipes that need a lighter oil.

TAMARI/SOY SAUCE: Many of the more elaborate recipes in the vegan world use a little bit of tamari or soy sauce, so it's a great staple to have. These are great for simple sauces, using sparingly over rice or quinoa, or accenting dressings. The low-sodium version tastes the same, so aim for that, if possible.

BALSAMIC VINEGAR/RICE WINE VINEGAR: Both of these vinegars have a distinctive and rich flavor, and can really add dimension to a ton of recipes.

BLACKSTRAP MOLASSES: This is a staple of the young vegan diet, because it's very high in iron and is a great way to get iron into small tummies by way of a little bit drizzled over oats, for example.

AGAVE NECTAR: Because many vegans don't use honey (it's an animal by-product), agave nectar is a great substitute to have on hand, and it's got a lower glycemic index, making it a healthier choice as well. Agave can be used in vegan dressings and sauces for a touch of sweetness, but it's also a perfect substitute for honey or sugar for almost any baking; Mayim even uses it to make veganized honey cake! Agave nectar is sweeter to taste than sugar or honey, so use ¾ cup of agave per 1 cup of honey or sugar called for in a recipe.

MAPLE SYRUP: Also used as a great sweetener; a little goes a long way. Can be used in small amounts to sweeten the CHILI on PAGE 152, for example, and is also a smart addition to dressings and sauces for sweetness that's not the processed refined sugar kind.

NUTRITIONAL YEAST: This is one of those things that you first hear of and think sounds crazy. Nutritional yeast is different than the yeast you use to make bread, and it's also different than brewer's yeast. Nutritional yeast is responsible for some of vegans' favorite "cheesy" recipes and it can be used to taste in mac and cheese dishes, sauces, and dips. Perhaps most delightfully, it can be sprinkled over KALE CHIPS (see PAGE 108) for a "cheesy" flavor.

KETCHUP: A must have for anyone with a small child, and you know why: kids will eat anything if they can dip it in ketchup. Or close to anything. Look for a corn syrup–free ketchup, if you can.

PREPARED DRESSINGS: There are many amazing choices of vegan dressings on the market. Obviously, we will share with you in this book some of our favorite do-it-yourself recipes, but having a bottle of vegan ranch, honey-mustard, Thousand Island, or Caesar dressing in your refrigerator makes for fun dipping, and salads that beg to be eaten.

JAM: Many people make their own jam, but if you buy, check for one that doesn't contain corn syrup, if possible.

Baking Staples

Here are some classic pantry items we recommend, from baking staples that we don't use as often but that are important to have in the house, to the basic grains and seeds that form the basis for a well-rounded vegan diet. In addition to vanilla extract, unsweetened cocoa powder, salt, baking pow-

der, and baking soda, here are some honorable pantry mentions.

FLOUR: White, whole wheat, and regular or whole wheat pastry: as there tends to be a healthier emphasis in vegan baking overall, whole wheat flour is often called for. Pastry flour makes for especially flaky and delicate desserts and pastries, which can be especially important because vegan recipes don't have eggs and achieving the right consistency of the batter can be the difference between yummy and yucky.

SUGAR: It's a good idea to have both white and brown, although a lot of vegan recipes lean heavier on the brown sugars. Sugar replacements, such as agave nectar (discussed on page 54) and Sucanat, are also options that can be good to stock up on, although they may be harder to locate in general.

EGG REPLACER: If you take out eggs from a recipe, you've got to put something in their place. In many recipes, a mashed banana or ¼ cup of applesauce does the trick with barely any difference in taste or consistency. (This is especially true for such things as sweet breads, muffins, and "fruity" baking.) For nonfluffy recipes, the following combination works great and is the most readily available: stir together 1 teaspoon of baking powder, 1 tablespoon of water, and 2 tablespoons of canola oil. However for more complicated breads and the real "binding power" that an egg provides, you'll want to have a commercial powdered egg replacer in your pantry. These are typically made from potato starch and some chemicals that, when combined with water, get fluffy and thick and make almost any recipe possible without the eggs. We like Ener-G, but several good brands are now available. As one box of egg replacer contains the equivalent of over one hundred eggs and it costs significantly less than buying eggs, we consider a good egg replacer a very wise decision for your wallet, your planet, and all of those sweet chickens out there who would prefer to keep their eggs.

CHOCOLATE CHIPS: Not only are vegan chocolate chips excellent for baking, but sometimes certain moms have doled out a few chocolate chips to get them through particularly difficult times. But never a lot. And never as a habit. And never with a spoonful of peanut or almond butter. It just might be good to have some on hand. You know; theoretically. For those tough times.

Spice Cabinet

There's nothing in particular that a vegan spice cabinet should have, but we want to give honorable mentions to the spices and herbs we tend to use and cook with the most.

SESAME SEEDS: A surprisingly terrific source of calcium, iron, and lignans, which have a cholesterol-lowering property. Sesame seeds are fun over salads, in dressings, and even in breads and cookies.

SALT: Use sea salt for grinding over food, kosher style for texture, and conventional salt for baking.

CINNAMON, GARLIC POWDER, OREGANO, AND CUMIN: Cumin is very popular in Middle Eastern cooking, and it's also used in a lot of vegan recipes. On its own, it's quite strong, but in the right dressing or sauce, it provides a really rich flavor.

Gadgets and Things

You can be a successful and excellent cook without most gadgets out there today, but here's a list of the most-used kitchen supplies which can enhance

PACKAGED SNACKS

There are going to be times when you can't make homemade granola bars, the last apple's gone mushy, and the carrot sticks are wilted. Here are some of our favorite snacks that we eat and offer sparingly (and preferably when coupled with a protein, such as nut butter, or followed with fruit or veggies for added nutrients!):

CORN CAKES/RICE CAKES: These are especially good for small hands, and as palates get more advanced, you can add nut butter or jam. (Because corn is a common allergen, many wait until after 12 months to introduce it to infants, so make sure to be careful about taking note of when you try it for the first time and know the signs of allergic reaction, which can range from stomach upset to fussiness to diarrhea to respiratory and asthmatic problems. If you have any questions, be sure to consult with your pediatrician.)

GRANOLA BARS: Most of the processed "mainstream" bars contain corn syrup and a bunch of chemicals you don't need. As you'll see on PAGE 66, making granola bars and energy bars is not terribly hard, but if you do want to have some of the store-bought kind in your pantry, try to choose some of the raw brands out there, which tend to be lighter on chemicals and heavier on nutrition.

CRACKERS (A FEW VARIETIES): It's important to have crackers around for spreading things on; it just makes snacks more fun when kids especially have a variety to choose from. Again, keep an eye on ingredients (the fewer, the better) and aim for sugar- and corn syrup–free, as much as possible.

POPCORN: Always wonderful to have on hand for a quick snack.

your ability to make and prepare healthy and fun vegan food without a lot of stress.

1. RIDICULOUSLY POWERFUL HIGH-POWERED BLENDER: This is one of those "wish list" items that you won't ever regret putting on your wish list. The ability to blend greens into smoothies will significantly change your life and the life of anyone who tastes your smoothies. A high-powered blender, such as a Vitamix, has an incredibly powerful motor and blade, and can make pesto, soups, and even nut butter from raw nuts in incredibly fast time. This is a wonderful investment that will stay with you for many, many years of happy cooking. A high-powered blender can be pricey, but you'll use it every day. Really.

2. HANDHELD IMMERSION BLENDER/CHOPPER/MIXER: This inexpensive tool is great for blending soups and easily chopping and blending nuts, pastes, and veggie burger mixes. Many of us who own a food processor have found it pretty much unnecessary since investing in a simple handheld immersion gadget. Processors are still great, though, for shredding large amounts of potatoes and onions for LATKES, as we discuss on PAGE 129.

Basics

SIMPLE, STURDY SET OF SAUCEPANS/SKILLETS: The basics will do you just fine here. Mayim really loves her cast-iron cookware for its ease and durability. Many people budget over the course of several years to afford a few strong pans they love.

STRONG, STURDY CHEF'S KNIFE: Will make all of your cooking smoother, faster, and safer. This is another gadget worth investing in for years of culinary pleasure.

CUTTING BOARD: Get one you love; as you won't be working with meat, you don't need to worry about disinfecting, but you do want a strong cutting board that can be cleaned well. Bamboo ones are nice, but to be honest, whatever you like best is fine.

STRONG WOODEN SPOONS

DURABLE GARLIC PRESS

WHISK

SET OF MEASURING CUPS AND SPOONS: We prefer metal rather than plastic.

SET OF STURDY BAKING SHEETS

Parchment paper

Pastry brush: For oiling baking and cooking surfaces (we prefer these to more expensive cans or spray bottles).

Set of stacking glass bowls: Inexpensive, easy to clean, and great for both preparing food and serving food.

Here are some other kitchen honorable mentions:

Small bowls: For dipping things into; Ramekins are also a great choice and can be found at flea markets or thrift stores. They don't all need to match, but they should be indestructible, cute, and colorful, if possible. Thrift stores are also great for picking up an unmatched set of plates and bowls for small hands, and sometimes an eye-catching plate or bowl is just the thing to make mealtime or snacktime extra fun.

Tiny cute toothpicks or metal toothpicks: These turn any food into fun: again, this is all about presentation and if you find a set of metal toothpicks with cute characters on them, we guarantee your child will eat more healthy things using those toothpicks than they would without.

Mason jars: These are not only great for canning jams and such; they are also wonderful as drinking glasses, as they are nearly indestructible, easy for small hands to hold onto, and easy to clean.

Stainless-steel and glass storage containers: Better than plastic and easy to find—you can scour the clearance sales at kitchen supply stores or thrift stores to find miscellaneous containers. Who really cares if you don't have a full matching set of every kind of storage container? Certainly not us!

CHAPTER 5

Breakfast

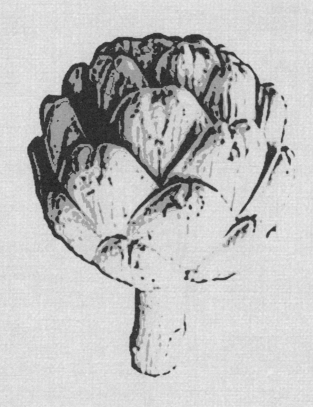

Outrageous Granola

MAKES 5 CUPS GRANOLA

Oats are a nutritious and satisfying way to start the day. This granola combines oats, nuts, and just the right amount of sweetness. You can be flexible with the types and amounts of all of the ingredients, depending on your taste preferences. It can be stored for up to a month in an airtight container.

Nonstick cooking spray

3 cups rolled oats

1 cup almonds, pecans, or your favorite nuts, chopped

1 cup dried fruit (any combination of cranberries, golden raisins, apricots, dates, cherries, and blueberries)

1 tablespoon vanilla extract

1 tablespoon ground cinnamon

½ teaspoon salt

⅓ cup packed brown sugar

1 cup maple syrup

1. Preheat the oven to 325°F. Spray a large, nonstick baking sheet with cooking spray.
2. Mix the remaining ingredients, except the dried fruit, together in a large bowl. Transfer to the baking sheet.
3. Bake for 35 to 45 minutes, until the granola starts to brown, stirring once halfway through the baking time.
4. Remove from the oven and let cool completely on the baking sheet. Mix in the dried fruit.

Green Smoothie

We think vegan breakfasts are best served smoothie-style, and this is a great starter smoothie. It's a perfect mix of sweet and healthy, with banana and pineapple for sweetness and hearty greens to give nutritional punch and vibrant color. Feel free to add other fruits and veggies and experiment.

2 bananas
1 cup spinach or kale leaves
½ cup frozen pineapple chunks
Handful of ice
2 cups water, nondairy milk, or juice (depending on your desired consistency)
1 tablespoon maple syrup
1 tablespoon flaxseed oil, or 1 avocado, peeled and pitted (optional)

1. Puree all the ingredients in a blender until smooth.

Peanut Butter Smoothie

MAKES TWO 1-CUP SERVINGS

This simple smoothie is ideal for the most finicky of palates. Protein-rich nut butter and banana combine for a rich, delicious way to start the day.

2 bananas
⅔ cup peanut butter (or half cup sunflower butter)
2 tablespoons maple syrup
1 cup rice milk
1 cup spinach leaves (optional)

1. Puree all the ingredients in a blender until smooth. You can also add 1 cup spinach leaves for more nutrients and flavor.

Fruity Oatmeal Smoothie

MAKES FOUR 1-CUP SERVINGS

This is one of the simplest and most tasty smoothies you can make. It's great if you need a quick breakfast on the run.

2½ cups nondairy milk
2 tablespoons quick oats
1 banana
½ cup fresh strawberries, hulled

1. Puree all the ingredients in a blender until smooth.

Rainbow Smoothie

MAKES FOUR 1-CUP SERVINGS

The goal of this smoothie is to have each color of the rainbow represented. With the following ingredients, you are getting a healthy dose of beta-carotene, vitamin C, potassium, calcium, iron, and tons of antioxidants. Measurements can vary, depending on what flavors you like best.

½ cup frozen or fresh strawberries or raspberries
1 orange, peeled, seeded, and sectioned
1 banana or 1 cup frozen pineapple chunks
1 cup spinach or kale leaves
½ cup frozen or fresh blueberries
Handful of ice
½ to 1 cup nondairy milk, preferably rice milk

1. Puree all the ingredients in a blender until smooth.

Fruity Oatmeal Muffins

MAKES 12 MUFFINS

Kids love a snack they can hold in their hands, and these nutritious and hearty muffins are not only kid-friendly, but easy to prepare. Add dried fruit or get creative with choco-late chips or nuts. Although they're perfect for breakfast with a little jam, you might find that these muffins become your go-to snack for any time of day.

1¼ cups rolled oats
¾ cup oat flour (run rolled oats through the blender until finely ground)
2 tablespoons potato starch
1 tablespoon baking powder
½ teaspoon ground cinnamon
½ teaspoon salt
¼ teaspoon ground nutmeg
¾ cup prunes or raisins, chopped
½ cup packed light brown sugar
½ cup vegetable oil
Egg replacer equivalent of 1 egg
1 cup unsweetened applesauce

1. Preheat the oven to 400°F. Place muffin-cup liners in twelve muffin cups.
2. Combine the oats, oat flour, potato starch, baking powder, cinnamon, salt, nut-meg, prunes or raisins, and brown sugar in a large bowl.
3. In a small bowl, beat the oil and the egg replacer until blended. Add the apple-sauce and stir until blended. Pour into the dry ingredients and stir until just blended.
4. Divide the batter among the prepared muffin cups and bake for 20 minutes, or until a wooden toothpick inserted into the center comes out clean. Let cool for 5 minutes in the pan set on a wire rack.

Super Energy Bars,
a.k.a. Raisin Apricot Bars

MAKES 12 BARS

So many granola bars are full of additives and preservatives, so we came up with a healthy homemade alternative. The base is whole wheat flour and oats, and you can tailor the nuts, dried fruits, and chocolate chip amounts to your taste. These bars are packed with energy-inspiring ingredients, and they can be cut into any shape. Not only does our version pack a more nutritious punch than commercial bars, they are definitely less expensive, too.

Canola cooking spray or 1 tablespoon canola oil
1 cup whole wheat flour
1 cup rolled oats
½ teaspoon sea salt
¼ cup vegetable oil
½ cup walnuts, finely chopped
½ cup raw pumpkin seeds, chopped
½ cup raisins, finely chopped
½ cup pitted prunes, finely chopped
1 cup dried apricots, finely chopped
1 tablespoon grated orange zest
1 cup vegan chocolate chips (optional)

1. Preheat the oven to 350°F. Grease an 8-inch square pan with canola cooking spray or the canola oil.
2. In a large bowl, mix the flour, oats, salt, and oil with your hands. Add the nuts, seeds, raisins, prunes, and apricots. Mix well. Add the orange zest and ¼ cup of water and mix until well combined. Add more water to bind, if necessary.
3. Spread out the mixture in the prepared pan and bake for 30 minutes. Remove from the oven, let cool completely in the pan, and cut into twelve bars.

Pancake Batter

MAKES 12 SMALL PANCAKES; SERVES 4

Vegan pancakes are hard to find in restaurants, so making them at home is a treat, especially when you hide nutritious and hearty ingredients and no one's the wiser. Whip up a few batches of the dry ingredients and store in an airtight container, then add the wet ingredients for easy pancakes any day of the week.

Nonstick cooking spray or vegan margarine, for the pan
1½ cups white whole wheat flour, or all-purpose or whole wheat flour
½ cup rolled oats
1 tablespoon baking powder
1 teaspoon salt
Egg replacer equivalent of 1 egg
1½ cups nondairy milk or water (or more, depending on the consistency desired)
2 tablespoons vegetable oil

1. Mix together the flour, oats, baking powder, salt, egg replacer, nondairy milk, and vegetable oil in a bowl. Do not overbeat, as the batter will get too thick.
2. Place a griddle pan over medium-high heat; oil the pan with nonstick cooking spray or a few tablespoons of vegan margarine. Pour out 4-inch circles or shapes. Cook for several minutes, until small bubbles form on the outer edge, and flip to lightly cook the other side, about 1 minute. Make sure the pan stays oiled for the remaining pancakes, adding oil by the tablespoon as the pan becomes dry.

Kitchen Tip

For an even healthier pancake, replace ½ cup of the flour with ½ cup of wheat germ or ground flaxseeds, or a combination of both.

French Toast

You don't need eggs or milk to make delicious French toast. This vegan version of every-one's favorite brunch dish is easy and scrumptious. Serve with maple syrup and fresh berries for a restaurant-worthy presentation.

2 to 3 ripe bananas, mashed, or ¼ cup smooth almond butter
1 cup plain unsweetened soy milk
¼ cup all-purpose flour
1 tablespoon nutritional yeast
1½ teaspoons ground cinnamon
1 teaspoon vanilla extract
3 tablespoons vegan margarine, for frying
About 6 slices of bread

1. In a large bowl, mix the bananas, soy milk, flour, nutritional yeast, cinnamon, and vanilla together until smooth.
2. Heat a griddle or large skillet on medium-high heat and melt 1 tablespoon of the margarine in the pan. Dip two bread slices into the banana mixture and then fry for 2 to 3 minutes on each side, until golden brown. Repeat with re-maining margarine and bread.

Cheese Melt

Grilled cheese has always been a kids' favorite, but this vegan version will remind you why grilled cheese can be so much fun for adults, too. Add olive tapenade for a mature flair, or keep it simple and serve with KALE CHIPS (PAGE 108), BRUSSELS SPROUTS CHIPS (PAGE 109), *or* OVEN-BAKED PARSNIP FRIES (PAGE 136) *for a well-balanced lunch or snack.*

2 slices whole-grain bread
2 teaspoons vegan margarine
2 slices nondairy cheese, Daiya preferred
Sliced tomato or sun-dried tomatoes
Sliced pickles
Sliced fresh or sautéed onion (see Kitchen Tip)
A leaf of kale, spinach, or any lettuce

1. Spread the margarine on both sides of the bread, about 1 teaspoon per slice. Top one slice with the cheese, tomato, pickles, onion, and the leafy green. Add the second slice of bread.
2. Over medium heat, grill the sandwich on both sides until the cheese melts and the bread is lightly browned.

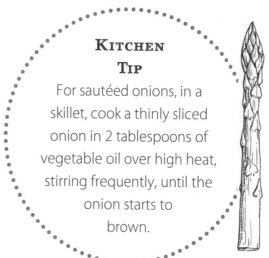

KITCHEN TIP

For sautéed onions, in a skillet, cook a thinly sliced onion in 2 tablespoons of vegetable oil over high heat, stirring frequently, until the onion starts to brown.

Breakfast Burrito

SERVES 4

A filling, tasty breakfast burrito is a great way to get your protein first thing in the morning. We've found that kids love burritos for breakfast, especially if they are easy to hold and you add some salsa for dipping!

2 tablespoons vegan margarine

½ yellow onion, chopped

½ teaspoon garlic, minced

1 red or green bell pepper, seeded and chopped

1 cup mushrooms, sliced

1 (14-ounce) can pinto or black beans, drained and rinsed

1 (14-ounce) package firm sprouted tofu, drained and diced into ½-inch cubes

⅛ teaspoon cayenne pepper

½ teaspoon freshly ground black pepper

1½ teaspoons turmeric

1 teaspoon salt

1 teaspoon olive oil

2 teaspoons maple syrup

1 tablespoon cider vinegar

1 cup chopped spinach

½ cup shredded vegan cheese, such as Daiya

4 large flour tortillas

½ cup salsa, for dipping (optional)

1. In a large skillet, heat the margarine over high heat. Sauté the onion, garlic, bell pepper, and mushrooms until soft, about 5 minutes. Add the beans and tofu, cayenne and black pepper, turmeric, salt, olive oil, maple syrup, and vinegar and cook for another 4 to 5 minutes. Gently add the spinach and cheese.

2. Warm the tortillas in the oven or microwave. Place the filling into the warmed tortillas and fold into burritos.

KITCHEN TIP

For variety, use the filling to make a quesadilla. Grill a tortilla, add the filling, and then place another tortilla on top to seal the deal. Use a pizza cutter to cut it up for easy eating.

Potato Hash

SERVES 4

Being vegan doesn't mean you have to miss out on diner-style foods, such as hearty hashes. This version uses packaged chorizo for a meaty flavor. Experiment by adding other diced vegetables to give it different flavors. You won't believe how tasty vegan hash can be!

2 large russet potatoes, peeled and diced
1 tablespoon canola oil
1 yellow onion, chopped
1 red or green pepper, seeded and chopped
1 teaspoon garlic, minced
½ cup fresh or frozen corn kernels
1 (14-ounce) can black beans, drained and rinsed
½ (12–ounce) package vegan chorizo

1. Place the potatoes in a large pot, cover with water, and bring to a boil. Lower the heat and simmer until tender, about 15 minutes. Drain and set aside.
2. In a large pan, heat the oil over high heat. Sauté the onion, pepper, and garlic until the onion is transparent, about 4 minutes. Add the potatoes and cook, stirring occasionally, until slightly browned, about 4 minutes. Add the chorizo and cook for 4 to 5 minutes, and then add the corn and beans and cook for another 2 to 3 minutes, stirring occasionally.

CHAPTER 6

Soups, Salads, and Sandwiches

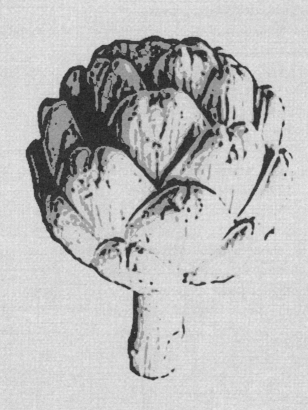

Butternut Squash Soup

SERVES 8

This is my Aunt Linda's recipe, and it's healthy, naturally sweet, and creamy. While it's great for autumn and winter meals, you can make it whenever squash is available. The hardest part is peeling the butternut squash, but after that, you just add everything to a pot, then simmer and blend it. We serve it with a hearty salad and crusty bread.

2 tablespoons vegan margarine

1 large white onion, chopped

1 garlic clove, minced

4 medium-size carrots, diced

2 celery stalks, leaves removed, sliced crosswise

1 large russet potato, peeled, and sliced or cubed

1 medium-size butternut squash, peeled, seeded, and diced (about 2 pounds)

3 (14.5-ounce) cans vegan vegetable stock

½ cup agave nectar or maple syrup

½ teaspoon dried thyme leaves, crushed

Salt and freshly ground pepper

Ground nutmeg (optional)

1. In a large pot, melt the margarine over medium heat. Stir in the onions and the garlic and cook until tender, 5 to 7 minutes.
2. Add all the remaining ingredients except the salt and the pepper, stir, and bring to a boil. Lower heat and simmer until all the vegetables are tender, about 45 minutes. Remove from heat and let cool slightly.
3. Working in small batches, transfer the soup to a blender or food processor and blend until smooth, or use an immersion blender in the pot.
4. Return the pureed soup to the pot and reheat over medium heat. Season to taste with salt and pepper and a pinch or two of ground nutmeg, if desired.

Cream of Carrot Soup

SERVES 8

It takes just a few ingredients to make this tasty carrot soup flavored with fresh dill.

2 pounds carrots, peeled and chopped
3 (14-ounce) cans of vegan vegetable stock
½ cup fresh dill, chopped
½ teaspoon salt
2 tablespoons sugar
¼ teaspoon freshly ground pepper
4 tablespoons (½ stick) vegan margarine
1 medium-size onion, chopped
¼ cup all purpose flour
2 cups nondairy milk, preferably soy

1. In a large stockpot, combine the carrots, vegetable stock, dill, sugar, salt, and pepper. Bring to a boil over high heat. Lower heat and simmer for 20 minutes or until the carrots are tender.
2. Meanwhile, melt the margarine in a large skillet over medium heat. Add the onion and cook for 4 to 5 minutes, until softened and starting to brown. Add the flour and cook, stirring for 3 minutes. Stir the cooked onions into the soup. Remove from heat and let cool slightly.
3. Working in small batches, transfer the soup to a blender or food processor and blend until smooth, or use an immersion blender in the pot. Return the pureed soup to the pot. Add the nondairy milk, stir, and reheat on medium for 5 minutes. Do not allow the soup to come to a boil.

Matzoh Ball Soup

MAKES 4 SERVINGS, 3 MATZOH BALLS EACH

Known as "Jewish penicillin," the immune-supporting properties of a classic chicken soup with matzoh balls can also be yours even if you're vegan. The rich broth is flavored with spices and tasty vegetables, and the fluffy matzoh balls are just as you'd expect with a classic nonvegan recipe. This recipe takes a little work, but the resulting flavor is worth it.

MATZOH BALLS

Egg replacer equivalent of 1 egg
1 (14-ounce) package firm sprouted tofu
¼ cup canola oil
2 (5-ounce) packages matzoh ball mix
1 teaspoon dried dill

VEGETABLE SOUP

2 tablespoons olive oil
½ cup carrots, chopped
½ cup celery, chopped
½ cup onions, chopped

BROTH

½ cup onions, chopped
½ cup celery, chopped
½ cup carrots, chopped
2 tablespoons vegan margarine
2 tablespoons onion powder
1 tablespoon garlic powder
1 tablespoon seasoned salt
2 tablespoons soy sauce
½ teaspoon dried poultry seasoning
Fresh flat-leaf parsley, chopped, for garnish

1. To make the matzoh balls, place the tofu and canola oil in a food processor and process until smooth. Add the egg replacer, the matzoh ball mix, and the dill, and blend well.
2. Transfer the mixture to a medium bowl. Cover and chill for at least 6 hours.
3. When ready, wet hands and roll the mixture into twelve balls the size of golf-balls. Return to the refrigerator, covered, until you are ready to cook them.
4. In a deep saucepan or stockpot, heat margarine over medium-low heat and cook the onions, celery, and carrots until the vegetables are soft, 5 to 7 minutes. Add 8 cups of water and onion powder, garlic powder, seasoned salt, poultry seasoning, and soy sauce. Simmer uncovered over medium-low heat for 30 minutes.
5. Strain the broth into a large pot and discard the vegetable pulp. Heat the broth over medium-high heat.
6. Heat olive oil over medium heat in a large skillet and saute carrots, celery, and onion for 10 minutes until tender. Add to pot of broth and bring to boil. Add matzoh balls and let simmer for 20 minutes. The balls will not increase in size but still will be fluffy and delicious. Garnish with chopped fresh parsley.

Mishmash Soup

This soup is what Mayim makes when she thinks she has nothing left in the house. It's an "everything but the kitchen sink" soup and can be as simple or complicated as you like. The main point is once you start with sautéed onion and garlic, it's hard to go wrong.

3 tablespoons olive oil

1 white onion, chopped

1 garlic clove, minced

3 cups veggies such as carrot, celery, bell pepper, or zucchini, diced

6 cups vegan vegetable stock

1 (14-ounce) can chopped tomatoes or 2 diced fresh tomatoes

1 (14-ounce) can beans, preferably kidney, white beans, or pinto

½ teaspoon each of three different dried herbs, such as basil, sage, thyme, rosemary, parsley, or oregano

½ bunch fresh dill and 1 bunch fresh parsley, bound with string

Salt and freshly ground pepper

Vegan crackers, toasted bread, croutons, or ½ cup cooked rice or quinoa

1. In a large pot, sauté onion and garlic in olive oil over medium heat until soft, about 5 minutes. Add the veggies and cook until they soften, 5 to 7 minutes. Add the vegetable stock, tomatoes, beans, dried herbs, and bundle of dill and parsley. Mix it all up and let it simmer for about 20 minutes, until the vegetables are tender. Season to taste with salt and pepper.
2. Remove herb bundle.
3. Serve with crackers, toasted bread, or croutons, or place cooked rice or quinoa in the bottom of each bowl and ladle the soup over it.

Minestrone

SERVES 8

One can never have too much minestrone soup. The herbs, the vegetables—and the inability to mess it up if you are missing one ingredient—make it a perfect soup when you need extra fluids and nutrients, or any time you crave a hearty Italian-style meal in a bowl. This version features squash for beautiful color and more nutritional punch.

2 tablespoons olive oil

1 yellow onion, chopped

2 celery stalks, chopped

2 medium-size carrots, peeled and chopped

1 teaspoon garlic, minced

6 cups vegan vegetable stock

One 2-pound butternut or Kabocha squash, peeled, seeded, and cut into 1-inch cubes; or 2 pounds russet potatoes, peeled and cut into 1-inch cubes

½ teaspoon dried oregano

½ teaspoon dried basil

1 bay leaf

1 sprig fresh thyme

1 (14-ounce) can crushed plum tomatoes

2 (14-ounce) cans white cannellini beans

½ pound green beans or zucchini, cut into 1-inch pieces

½ bunch kale, leaves only, cut into bite-sized pieces

3 cups slightly undercooked pasta (fusilli or penne)

Salt and freshly ground pepper

1. In a large pot, heat olive oil over high heat. Sauté the onions, celery, carrots, and garlic until soft, 4 to 5 minutes.
2. Add stock, squash, herbs, and tomatoes and simmer for 20 to 30 minutes. Add the white beans, green beans or zucchini, kale, and pasta and cook for a further 10 minutes. Season to taste with salt and pepper.

Tomato Soup with Israeli Couscous

SERVES 4–6

Soup is sometimes where great meal planning starts, especially with delicious and so-phisticated flavors like those you'll find in this Middle Eastern–inspired soup. The garlic and deceptively simple spices create a complex base. With the addition of couscous, this soup is a meal in itself.

2 tablespoons olive oil
1 onion, chopped
1 to 2 carrots, diced
1 (14-ounce) can chopped tomatoes
6 garlic cloves, roughly chopped
6¼ cups vegan vegetable stock
1 to 1½ cups uncooked Israeli couscous
2 to 3 mint sprigs, chopped, or several pinches of dried mint
¼ teaspoon ground cumin
¼ bunch fresh cilantro or about 5 sprigs, chopped
Salt and freshly ground pepper

1. Heat the olive oil in a large pan, add the onion and carrots, and cook over medium-low for about 10 minutes until softened. Add the tomatoes, half of the garlic, vegetable stock, couscous, mint, cumin, and cilantro.
2. Bring the soup to boil, add the remaining chopped garlic, then lower the heat slightly and simmer gently for 7 to 10 minutes, stirring occasionally, or until the couscous is just tender. Season to taste with salt and pepper.

Israeli Salad

SERVES 4

The key to this versatile salad is making sure all of the ingredients are diced the same size, and as small as possible, so the flavors really blend. Some people prefer more onion, less pickle, or more spice. For an extra kick, add another clove of minced garlic.

Israeli salad is made to be served with falafel in pita layered with hummus, but this salad is a great side dish with any meal.

6 small cucumbers, preferably Persian with thin skins

3 medium-size tomatoes

6 Israeli pickles

½ medium-size white onion

3 tablespoons olive oil

A squeeze of lemon, approximately
    1 tablespoon

½ teaspoon salt

½ teaspoon freshly ground black pepper

1. Dice the cucumber, tomato, pickles and onion into ¼- to ½-inch cubes and place in a large bowl.
2. Drizzle liberally with olive oil and a squeeze of lemon and sprinkle with salt and pepper to taste. Marinate for at least 2 hours covered in the fridge so the flavors can mingle.

KITCHEN TIP

Israeli pickles are typically found in most kosher markets. They are sometimes called cucumbers in brine, but dill pickles or bread and butter pickles won't taste right. This salad works without the pickle as well if you can't find any!

Simple Greens with Agave Mustard Dressing

Because it is an animal by-product, many vegans don't use honey. Mayim could not bear to eliminate her favorite honey mustard dressing from her life, so she created this version with agave nectar as a substitute. It's paired here with a simple romaine salad and homemade croutons, one of Mayim's specialties. This dressing is a winner even over vegetables, so make a little extra to use as a marinade.

Nonstick cooking spray

CROUTONS
3 to 4 cups cubed bread
¼ cup olive oil
1 tablespoon balsamic vinegar
½ teaspoon salt
¼ teaspoon freshly ground black pepper
2 teaspoons dried herbs, such as rosemary or oregano (optional)

AGAVE MUSTARD DRESSING
½ cup olive oil
3 tablespoons balsamic vinegar
1 tablespoon mustard (plain yellow, deli, or whatever you have on hand)
1 tablespoon agave nectar
1 garlic clove, minced
½ teaspoon salt
⅛ teaspoon freshly ground black pepper

1 bag or bunch romaine lettuce or spinach, or spring mix of greens
3 scallions, sliced

1. Preheat the oven to 350°F. Lightly spray a baking sheet with nonstick cooking spray.
2. To make the croutons, place the bread cubes in a bowl and drizzle generously with olive oil and balsamic vinegar. Sprinkle with salt and pepper. Add the herbs if you desire. Mix until well saturated and place on the baking sheet.
3. Toast in the oven until lightly browned, about 15 minutes, depending on the size of the cubes.
4. To make the salad dressing, place all the ingredients in a small bowl and mix vigorously with a fork or whisk. For a thicker and creamier dressing, combine the ingredients in a hand chopper or mini food processor and blend well.
5. To assemble the salad, place the lettuce and scallions in a large bowl. Add the croutons. The dressing will settle, so mix it again just before pouring it over the salad and croutons.

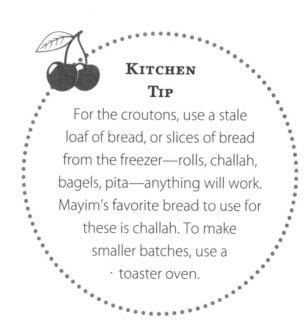

KITCHEN TIP

For the croutons, use a stale loaf of bread, or slices of bread from the freezer—rolls, challah, bagels, pita—anything will work. Mayim's favorite bread to use for these is challah. To make smaller batches, use a toaster oven.

Asian Salad Two Ways

SERVES 4

Chinese Chicken Salad was one of Mayim's favorite childhood dinners. This version can be enjoyed as a broccoli slaw or as a more traditional Asian-inspired salad, with a tangy rice vinegar-based dressing for both. Sesame seeds are a great source of minerals including calcium and iron, so this salad also packs a nutritional punch.

1. BROCCOLI SLAW

1 (12-ounce) bag broccoli slaw

1 (8-ounce) bag shelled edamame, cooked according to directions

⅓ cup slivered or chopped almonds

2 tablespoons sesame seeds

1. Mix broccoli, edamame and almonds in a large bowl. Stir in dressing (below). Sprinkle sesame seeds on top.

2. TRADITIONAL CHINESE NO-CHICKEN

5 cups Romaine or a combination or romaine and spinach

3 scallions, sliced

½ cup slivered or chopped almonds

1 (11-ounce) can drained Mandarin oranges

2 tablespoons sesame seeds

1. Mix lettuce, scallions, and oranges in a bowl. Stir in dressing (below). Sprinkle sesame seeds on top.

ASIAN DRESSING

½ cup sesame oil

¾ cup rice wine vinegar

3 tablespoons duck sauce (optional)

2 tablespoons agave nectar

1 tablespoon soy sauce

1. Whisk ingredients together in a small bowl and pour over broccoli slaw or salad. Toss to combine.

Sweet and Sour Cabbage Salad

SERVES 4

Mayim's grandmother loved making this salad because it mimicked the Hungarian pickled vegetables and salads of her childhood. The marinade is a balanced combination of sweet and sour. This salad will keep for several days in the refrigerator.

1 head cabbage, coarsely shredded
2 cucumbers, thinly sliced
3 carrots, thinly sliced
1 large onion, thinly sliced

MARINADE
½ cup white vinegar
½ cup sugar
¼ cup oil
4 tablespoons water
1 ½ teaspoon salt

1. Place the cut vegetables in a large bowl and mix together.
2. In a medium bowl, mix the marinade ingredients together and pour over the vegetables. Marinate for at least 2 hours in the refrigerator.

Potato Salad

Looking for dish to bring to a barbeque, to amp up the plant-based options? This old-fashioned creamy version of America's favorite side dish will shock non-vegans with its rich and authentic taste. Add more diced vegetables to make it a heartier meal, or serve as is as a side dish and watch it disappear.

2 pounds Russet potatoes, unpeeled
½ (16-ounce) bag frozen peas, defrosted
½ red onion, finely chopped
3 stalks celery, finely chopped

DRESSING
1 cup vegan mayonnaise
1 tablespoon white vinegar
1 tablespoon mustard, preferably deli style
1 teaspoon salt
½ teaspoon freshly ground black pepper

1. Place the potatoes in a large pot, cover with water, add 2 teaspoons salt, and bring to boil. Simmer until tender but not soft, about 14 minutes. Remove from heat, drain, cut in half and let cool a bit.
2. Dice the potatoes into bite-size pieces and place in large bowl with the peas, onion and celery.
3. In a small bowl, combine dressing ingredients and pour over the potatoes and veggies. Stir to combine and let cool in the fridge for at least 1 hour.

Build-Your-Own Taco Salad

SERVES 4

Many parents get tired of toddler-aged kids picking apart their meals to separate things they like from things they don't. Mayim's solution is this healthy and delicious dinner with everything diced the same size so that kids won't be tempted to pick things out.

This salad can be assembled beforehand or with the help of any especially finicky eaters, but don't be surprised if you assemble it, sprinkle tortilla chips on top, add a dollop of vegan sour cream and salsa, and watch it all disappear, with no picking apart at all!

8 cups spinach or romaine, finely chopped

2 large tomatoes, diced

1 (15-ounce) can black beans, drained

1 (12–ounce) bag frozen corn, thawed and drained

1 red onion, finely chopped

3 tablespoons cilantro, chopped (optional)

2 cups seitan strips, sautéed in 2 Tablespoons olive oil (optional)

2 cups tortilla chips or corn chips

Vegan sour cream

Barbecue sauce or salsa

Vegan ranch dressing (optional)

1. Combine the vegetables and seitan, if using, in a large bowl and toss.
2. Crumble chips on top. Put out the sour cream, dressings and sauces—whatever you have on hand—and let everyone choose whichever they want.

Three-Bean Salad

Anyone raised in the United States between 1950 and today has probably experienced the beauty of a canned Three-Bean Salad. This homemade version is a colorful side dish to pair with veggie dogs or veggie burgers for summertime barbeques. We prefer to use agave nectar rather than sugar for a lower glycemic index, but you just want to be sure the salad is sweet enough to counter the tang of vinegar. Add canned corn kernels or substitute other kinds of cooked beans, such as lima beans, if you like.

1 cup cooked or canned kidney beans
1 cup cooked or canned string beans
1 cup cooked or canned wax beans
1 cup onion, diced
½ cup celery, chopped
½ cup green pepper, chopped
½ cup pimento or roasted red pepper, chopped
1 cup vegetable oil
2 cups white vinegar
1 cup sugar
1 teaspoon salt (or more to taste)
½ teaspoon freshly ground black pepper
2 tablespoons fresh chopped dill

1. Combine the oil, vinegar, sugar, salt, pepper, and dill in a bowl. Pour over the beans, onion, celery, green pepper, and pimento. Let marinate in the refrigerator at least 1 hour before serving.

NOTE: *This salad can be made in advance. It keeps well for 3 days.*

Moroccan Vegetable Salad

An easy and fresh alternative to traditional green salads, this chilled North African–inspired dish combines potato, bell peppers, cucumbers, and olives with a light and tangy vinaigrette. Simple to prepare, it's great to double or triple for potlucks or group meals. Serve with the salad spread out on a large platter to let the colors and shapes of the ingredients shine. Make extra dressing to reinvigorate leftovers the next day. For a pretty variation, serve the salad garnished with sliced or diced cooked beets.

1 large cucumber, thinly sliced

2 cold, boiled potatoes, sliced

1 each red, yellow and green bell peppers, seeded and thinly sliced

$^2/_3$ cup pitted olives

Salt (optional)

3 garlic cloves, chopped

3 scallions, sliced or 1 red onion, finely chopped

4 tablespoons olive oil

1 tablespoon white wine vinegar

Juice of ½ lemon

1 tablespoon chopped fresh mint leaves

1 tablespoon chopped fresh cilantro leaves

1. Arrange the cucumber, potato and pepper slices, and the pitted olives on a serving plate or in a dish.
2. Season with salt, if you like. (Olives tend to be very salty so you may not wish to add any extra salt.)
3. Sprinkle the garlic, onions, olive oil, vinegar, and lemon juice over the salad. Chill for at least 1 hour. Before serving, sprinkle with the chopped mint leaves and cilantro leaves.

Coleslaw Two Ways

SERVES 4

Here's another side dish that many vegans think they have to give up when they go veg, but with vegan mayonnaise, you can still enjoy coleslaw. Don't be limited by cabbage alone; add shredded carrots for a colorful take. Try the vinaigrette variation for a lighter, tart option.

1. CREAMY COLESLAW

¼ cup vegan mayonnaise

1 tablespoon apple cider vinegar

4 cups cabbage, sliced (you can use bagged from the store)

1 teaspoon salt

½ teaspoon freshly ground black pepper

¼ bunch cilantro, chopped

¼ red onion, thinly sliced

1. In a large bowl, mix the mayonnaise, vinegar, salt, and pepper. Add the cabbage and massage to coat. Mix in the cilantro and onions.

2. COLESLAW WITH VINAIGRETTE

¼ cup canola or vegetable oil

¼ cup cider vinegar

¼ cup brown sugar

¼ teaspoon salt

¼ teaspoon dry mustard

4 cups cabbage, sliced (you can use bagged from the store)

1. In a large bowl, mix the oil, vinegar, brown sugar, mustard, and salt. Add the cabbage and massage to coat.

Quinoa Salad with Veggies and Herbs

SERVES 6

When Mayim first became vegan, she saw a recipe in a magazine for barley salad with herbs. She substituted the barley with quinoa, a high protein seed from South America that is incredibly versatile, inexpensive, and easy to make. The result is one of her favorite dishes to bring to potlucks. You can prepare it with almost any vegetables and herbs you have on hand. The secret is to use a generous amount of the dressing and let it set for a few hours before serving.

1 cup quinoa, rinsed
½ cup scallions, green parts only, chopped
½ cup red bell pepper, seeded and diced
½ cup fresh or frozen peas, thawed
¼ cup fresh flat-leaf parsley, chopped
⅓ cup fresh basil leaves, chopped
2 tablespoons fresh mint leaves
¼ cup canola oil
1 garlic clove, minced
1 tablespoons freshly squeezed lemon juice
Salt and freshly ground black pepper

1. In a medium saucepan, combine the quinoa and 2 cups water over high heat. Bring to a boil. Lower the heat to low and simmer, covered, until all the water is absorbed, 10 to 15 minutes. Drain and set aside.
2. In a large bowl, combine scallions, red pepper, peas, parsley, basil and mint. Toss in the cooked quinoa.
3. In a small bowl, whisk together the oil, garlic, and lemon juice. Season to taste with salt and pepper, then toss into the salad, stirring to combine well. Let stand for 1 hour for flavors to set.

Rainbow Cabbage Salad
with Tahini-Lemon Dressing

SERVES 4

This colorful salad is delicious as a main course or side dish. The nutritional punch of colors makes it full of beta-carotene, calcium, and a bevy of vitamins. Arrange the ingredients alongside one another and drizzle with the dressing, or mix them all together for a mixed-up delicious rainbow of a salad.

3 tablespoons toasted sesame or sunflower seeds
6 cups red cabbage, roughly chopped (about ¼ large cabbage)
1 large carrot, peeled then shaved (using the peeler) into 2–3-inch strips
3 celery stalks, leaves removed, chopped
1 red bell pepper, seeded and thinly sliced
2 handfuls of fresh flat-leaf parsley, finely chopped

TAHINI-LEMON DRESSING
4 ounces tahini
1 garlic clove
Juice of ½ lemon
Pinch of cayenne pepper

½ teaspoon salt
¼ teaspoon freshly ground black pepper

1. Preheat the oven to 325°F. Using a rimmed baking sheet, toast the seeds for 8 to 10 minutes, watching closely. You can also use a toaster oven until the seeds start to darken, or sauté them without oil in a small pan until they brown and become fragrant, about 5 minutes. Remove and set aside.
2. Boil 8 cups of water while you chop the cabbage. Slice cabbage in half through the stem. Slice each half in half again and chop roughly. Place the chopped cabbage into a strainer over your sink and pour the boiling water over it. Rinse

quickly with cold water. Dry the cabbage roughly with a (dark-colored) hand towel or in a salad spinner.

3. In a large bowl, mix together the celery, pepper, cabbage, shaved carrot, and parsley.

4. Place all the dressing ingredients in a blender. Add enough water to make a dressing consistency. Add the dressing to the cabbage salad just before serving.

Americana Pasta Salad

SERVES 4

It's important to have vegan comfort food on hand, and this pasta salad with its rich creamy dressing will not disappoint. It's a perfect side dish for veggie burgers or veggie dogs, adding defrosted peas, corn, and carrots works well for more color and flavor.

CREAMY DRESSING
½ cup vegan mayonnaise
2 teaspoons sugar
2 teaspoons white vinegar
½ teaspoon prepared mustard
½ teaspoon salt
Freshly ground black pepper

2 cups cooked pasta, cooled slightly
¼ cup celery, chopped
¼ cup onion, chopped
½ cup peas, or a mixture of peas and carrots, thawed

1. In a small bowl, whisk vegan mayonnaise, sugar, vinegar, mustard, and salt. Add pepper to taste.
2. In a large bowl, combine pasta, celery, onion, and peas or peas and carrots. Add dressing and toss to coat.

Corn and Black Bean Salad

SERVES 4

This creamy salad is great as a side dish and it's full of protein. Mayim got this recipe from her friend Cara Paiuk, who is a writer and also a creator of amazing vegan cheeses in her spare time. Kids seem to love this combination of flavors and textures, and you can substitute pinto or garbanzo beans if you don't have black beans on hand.

1 (14-ounce) can corn
½ (14-ounce) can black beans, drained and rinsed
1 (14-ounce) can hearts of palm, cut into ¼-inch rounds

CREAMY DRESSING
3 tablespoons vegan mayonnaise
2 teaspoons freshly squeezed lemon juice
1 teaspoon dry dill
1 teaspoon garlic powder
½ medium-size shallot, minced
Generous pinch of sugar

1. Combine the corn, beans, and hearts of palm in a large bowl.
2. Whisk all the dressing ingredients together in a small bowl. Add to the salad and toss.

Quinoa Mango Salad

SERVES 4

Quinoa salads are a staple in many Jewish homes during Passover, when grains are not consumed for eight days and quinoa takes center stage. This one is light, a little tangy, and full of protein from the quinoa and the nuts. It keeps for 2 to 3 days and is perfect as a main course or a side dish.

1½ cups quinoa, rinsed
6 basil leaves, finely chopped
3 sprigs fresh cilantro, gently torn
⅓ cup red onion, minced
½ or 1 firm mango, peeled and diced into ⅛-inch pieces
2 tablespoons olive oil
¾ teaspoon fine sea salt
1 tablespoon plus 1 teaspoon freshly squeezed lime juice
¼ cup ground cashews

1. In a medium saucepan, combine the quinoa and 3 cups of water over high heat. Bring to a boil. Lower the heat to low and simmer, covered, until all the water is absorbed, 10 to 15 minutes. Drain and set aside.
2. In a large bowl, combine basil, cilantro, red onion, and mango with the quinoa.
3. Combine the olive oil, salt, lime juice, and ground cashews in a small bowl and whisk together. Season to taste with salt and pepper and pour over the salad.

Quinoa Burgers

SERVES 4

In this age of substitute faux meats, many people find that vegan burgers try too hard to be meaty. This quinoa burger makes a lighter veggie burger to slide into a bun, wrap, or pita. Mashed potato binds the quinoa, keeping the burger whole. With the condiments of your choosing, this burger will not disappoint.

1 large russet potato, peeled and diced
1 cup uncooked quinoa, rinsed
½ teaspoon ground cumin
½ teaspoon dried oregano
2 garlic cloves, minced
½ teaspoon salt
¼ teaspoon freshly ground black pepper
1 tablespoon vegetable oil

1. Preheat the oven to 350°F. Place the potato in a small saucepan and cover with water. Heat to a boil over high heat, and simmer for 12 minutes or until tender. Drain.
2. In a medium saucepan, combine the quinoa and 3 cups water over high heat. Bring to a boil. Lower the heat to low and simmer, covered, until all the water is absorbed, 10 to 15 minutes. Drain and set aside.
3. In a large bowl, mix the cooked potato and quinoa with all the remaining ingredients except the oil. Shape the mixture into four 3-inch diameter patties and set aside.
4. In a 10-inch skillet, heat the oil over high heat. Place each patty in the oil and fry until browned on both sides, about 2 minutes. Remove the patties and place them on an oven-safe dish. Pat the patties with a paper towel to remove the excess oil.
5. Bake for 10 minutes.

Vietnamese Banh Mi
with Do Chua and Sweet Sauce

When Mayim was a student at UCLA, students lined up for blocks for the campus' finest Vietnamese sandwiches. She never got to taste the non-vegan version, but she created her own that rivals that little restaurant from her college days. The toasted baguette, the crunchy tart carrot and parsnip salad of do chua, and the sweet sauce add up to a hearty sandwich that's big on flavor and color.

DO CHUA
2 large carrots, peeled and cut into matchsticks

1 pound daikon radish, peeled and cut into matchsticks

1 teaspoon salt

½ cup sugar

1½ cups white vinegar

SWEET SAUCE
½ cup rice vinegar

¼ cup light brown sugar, packed

2 tablespoons soy sauce

2 garlic cloves, peeled and smashed

1 teaspoon crushed red pepper flakes

1 baguette or loaf French bread

Vegan mayonnaise

1 (14-ounce) container firm tofu, drained and cut into strips

1. To make the do chua, place the carrots and daikon in a medium bowl and sprinkle with the salt. Knead vegetables for 2 to 3 minutes to expel their water. Soon some liquid will pool at the bottom of the bowl. Stop kneading when the vegetables are wilted. Drain them in a colander and wash under cold, running water. Press the vegetables gently to drain the extra water. Place in a quart-size jar.

2. Mix the sugar, vinegar and 1 cup of warm water in a small bowl. Stir until the sugar is dissolved. Pour this liquid over the vegetables, covering them completely.

3. Refrigerate for at least 1 hour before serving. Do chua will keep in the fridge for about 4 weeks.

4. To make the sweet sauce, combine all the ingredients in a small saucepan over high heat and bring to a boil. Lower the heat to medium and simmer, uncovered, for 10 minutes. Remove from the heat, let cool, remove the garlic cloves, and serve.

5. To make the banh mi, cut the baguette in half lengthwise into 4 to 5 pieces and toast. Spread vegan mayonnaise and dipping sauce on both sides. Lay 3 strips of tofu on each sandwich. Add do chua, and more dipping sauce, if desired.

Dilled Chickpea Burger with
Spicy Yogurt Sauce

SERVES 6

No one will ever know these burgers are made of chickpeas, unless you tell them. Shallots, chickpeas, tahini, and spices are combined and sautéed to crisp perfection for one of the most satisfying veggie burgers we've tasted. Here we've stuffed them into pita pockets and doused them with yogurt sauce, but they're just as wonderful with ketchup and mustard, or raw onion and a little hummus and ISRAELI SALAD (PAGE 81). *These are thinner patties that should be cooked until crisp. Handle them as little as possible, and let them cook well on the first side before flipping.*

YOGURT SAUCE
1 cup plain vegan yogurt
2 garlic cloves, peeled and minced
½ teaspoon curry powder
¼ teaspoon cayenne pepper

1 (15-ounce) can chickpeas, well-drained and rinsed
⅓ cup fresh dill, finely chopped
½ cup shallots, minced
2 tablespoons plain dry bread crumbs
2 tablespoons freshly squeezed lemon juice
2 tablespoons tahini
½ teaspoon salt
¼ teaspoon coarsely ground black pepper
¼ teaspoon ground cumin
About ¼ cup vegetable oil, for oiling the pan
6 pita pockets or buns

1. To make the yogurt sauce, place all the ingredients in a small bowl and stir until blended thoroughly.
2. To make the burger, lightly mash half of the chickpeas in a medium bowl. Add the dill, shallots, bread crumbs, and lemon juice and mix well.

3. In a food processor, combine the remaining chickpeas, tahini, salt, pepper and cumin until smooth. Add to the mashed chickpeas, mix well, and form into six to eight patties.

4. Oil a 12-inch skillet over medium heat and cook the burgers until very crispy and dark golden on both sides, about 6 minutes. Don't flip them too much! Drain on paper towels or brown paper bags on a wire rack.

5. Stuff the patties in pita pockets. Drizzle with yogurt sauce.

Vegan Reuben Sandwiches

MAKES 4 SANDWICHES

It's hard to give up your favorite sandwich when you make the decision to eat plant-based foods, but this Reuben recipe will make you forget you ever doubted your decision. We've re-created the flavor of a classic deli Ruben with ingredients and spices that mimic the original to a T. Grilling the rye bread makes all the difference, so don't skip that step!

THOUSAND ISLAND DRESSING
⅓ cup vegan mayonnaise

2 tablespoons ketchup

3 tablespoons dill pickles, diced

SAUTÉED ONIONS
3 tablespoons vegetable oil

1 large yellow onion, thinly sliced

1 teaspoon garlic, minced

2 bay leaves

1½ teaspoons paprika

¾ teaspoon caraway seeds

¾ teaspoon dried dill

1 teaspoon salt

2 tablespoons cider vinegar

1 tablespoon tamari

¼ teaspoon freshly ground black pepper

8 slices vegan rye bread

8 slices vegan bacon

2 tablespoons vegan margarine

1 cup sauerkraut, drained

1. To make the dressing, combine all the ingredients in a small bowl.
2. To make the onions, heat the vegetable oil in a large skillet over medium heat. Add the onion and cook for 5 minutes, stirring occasionally. Stir in the garlic, bay leaves, paprika, caraway seeds, dill, salt, vinegar, tamari, and pepper. Add the water and simmer uncovered for 10 minutes, or until the liquid has evaporated. Remove the bay leaves.
3. Heat a large skillet over medium-high heat. Spread two slices of the bread with margarine. Grill in a small skillet, margarine side down, for 3 minutes on one side only. Repeat with the remaining slices of bread.
4. To assemble each sandwich, spread the dressing on the ungrilled sides of two slices of toast. Add the sauerkraut, two pieces of vegan bacon, and the sautéed onions.

Falafel

SERVES 6

Falafel tends to be a vegan favorite, since it is high in protein, easy to bind without egg, and delicious in a pita or on a plate with hummus and Israeli salad for a full meal. This falafel recipe captures the authentic flavors of a Middle Eastern delicacy. Because falafel is fried, serve it with enough side salads to give a nutritional balance, and make sure to drain the falafel well before serving so it stays light and crunchy. Mayin makes this for gluten-free friends by substituting gluten-free bread crumbs.

2 cups cooked or canned chickpeas, drained and rinsed
¼ cup bread crumbs
2–3 tablespoons superfine brown rice flour
1 medium-size onion, chopped
2 garlic cloves, minced
½ teaspoon baking powder
1 teaspoon ground cumin
1 teaspoon ground coriander
¼ teaspoon chipotle or cayenne pepper
¼ cup fresh flat-leaf parsley, chopped
½ teaspoon salt
Vegetable oil for frying

OPTIONAL ADDITIONS
Lettuce
Tomato, cucumber, and/or red onion, chopped
Tahini dressing
Hummus

1. Blend the chickpeas and bread crumbs in a food processor. Add the remaining ingredients and process until well combined and smooth.
2. Refrigerate for at least 30 minutes, then shape into golfball-size balls and flatten slightly.
3. Heat ½ inch of the oil in a cast-iron or other heavy pan until hot, but not so hot that smoke rises. Cook the patties in batches for 2½ to 3 minutes on each side until browned and crisp. Drain on paper towels or brown paper bags on a wire rack and serve with the accompaniments of your choice.

Build-Your-Own
Tofu Napa Cabbage Wraps

SERVES 4

We love meals that families can assemble on their own. Everyone gets what they want and nothing they don't. Kids will love the wrap-ability of napa cabbage, and parents will love the protein and healthy crunch of these wraps. We like serving this with quickly pickled Vietnamese vegetables (do chua) to add interest, and a little splash of sweet sauce makes these wraps something special: nutritious, fun, and so yummy.

1 (14-ounce) container firm tofu, drained and cut into strips
8 napa cabbage leaves
¼ cup peanuts, chopped
⅛ cup cilantro sprigs
¼ cup cooked rice noodles or crunchy chow mein noodles
1 cup DO CHUA (PAGE 98)
½ cup SWEET SAUCE (PAGE 98)

1. Place each ingredient or sauce in its own bowl for self-assembly.
2. For each wrap, place a strip of tofu in a cabbage leaf. Sprinkle with peanuts, cilantro, noodles, do chua, and drizzle with sweet sauce.

CHAPTER 7

Snacks, Sauces, and Dips

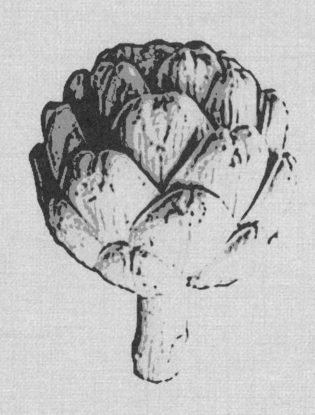

Kale Chips

Kale chips are one of the easiest, healthiest and most fun vegan snacks we can think of. These are great for parties, and when sprinkled with nutritional yeast, they are one of the most irresistible vegan snacks you'll ever taste.

2 bunches kale, stems removed, diced into 2- to 3-inch pieces
3 tablespoons olive oil
1 teaspoon sea salt
2 tablespoons nutritional yeast (optional)

1. Preheat the oven to 350°F. Place the kale pieces on two baking sheets and drizzle generously with olive oil, tossing to coat. Sprinkle with the sea salt and nutritional yeast, if using.
2. Bake, turning every 5 to 7 minutes, until browned and crunchy, almost burnt, but not burnt.

Brussels Sprouts Chips

Brussels sprouts chips take a bit more work to prep than kale chips, but the result is crunchy and delicious and rivals potato chips any day of the week.

1 pound brussels sprouts
3 tablespoons olive oil
1 teaspoon sea salt

1. Preheat the oven to 350°F. Remove the leaves of the brussels sprouts. This is tedious work, but it can be done. You want as many leaves as possible, and you may need to keep cutting away the stem as you get deeper into the sprout.
2. Place the leaves on a baking sheet and drizzle generously with olive oil, tossing to coat. Sprinkle with the sea salt. Bake, turning every 5 to 7 minutes, until browned and crunchy, almost burnt, but not burnt.

Guacamole

Avocados are a vegan's best friend, full of healthy fats, protein, and tons of vitamins. Here is Dr. Jay's simple recipe for nutritious and delicious guacamole for dipping, spreading, or eating straight from the bowl. Serve with chips, crackers, carrots, celery, jicama, and any vegetable good for dipping.

4 avocados, pitted
½ white onion, diced small
2 tablespoons fresh cilantro, chopped
Juice of 1 lime
1 teaspoon salt
1 small garlic clove, minced
1 medium-size tomato, diced

1. Scoop the avocado flesh into a bowl and mash. Add all the remaining ingredients, except the tomato. Stir to combine, adding the tomato last.

Raw Nut Cheese

One of the questions vegans get asked most often is, "But how do you live without cheese?" Now you can answer, "I don't." This versatile recipe for nut-based cheese will be delicious with whatever fresh or dried herbs you have in your kitchen or garden. It can be blended smooth like a pâté spread, or left a bit chunky to resemble and substitute for ricotta. No matter how you make it, this cheese will make you grateful that you don't have to miss the cheesy recipes you used to love.

1 cup raw cashews, almonds, or walnuts
1 tablespoon fresh basil
1 tablespoon fresh rosemary
1 tablespoon freshly squeezed lemon juice
1 teaspoon sea salt

1. Soak the nuts in water to cover. For cashews, soak overnight. For almonds or walnuts, 4 hours is enough. Drain.
2. Place the softened nuts in a blender and add the basil, rosemary, lemon juice, and salt. Mix until combined and smooth but not creamy.

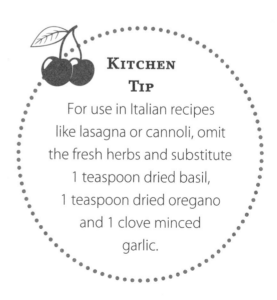

KITCHEN TIP

For use in Italian recipes like lasagna or cannoli, omit the fresh herbs and substitute 1 teaspoon dried basil, 1 teaspoon dried oregano and 1 clove minced garlic.

Mexican Bean Dip

MAKES 1 1/4 CUPS

Mayim's good friend Nancy introduced this bean dip into their circle of holistically minded moms years ago, and it was an instant hit. Who knew that cumin and soy sauce, when combined with beans, onion and garlic, could be so delicious? Serve this dip with cut up veggies, warm tortillas, or line burritos or tacos with it for a creative twist on re-fried beans.

1 tablespoon olive oil

¼ cup onion, chopped

1 garlic clove, minced

2 tablespoons celery, finely chopped

1½ cups cooked kidney or pinto beans, or 1 (14-ounce) can, drained and rinsed

¼ teaspoon soy sauce

¼ teaspoon ground cumin

⅛ teaspoon cayenne pepper (optional)

1. Heat the olive oil in a large skillet on medium heat, and sauté the onion, garlic, and celery until soft, about 5 minutes. Add the beans and seasonings, and stir until well mixed. Spoon into a blender or food processor and puree until smooth.

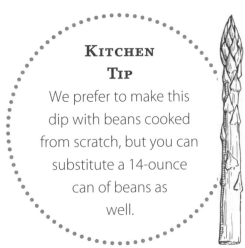

KITCHEN TIP

We prefer to make this dip with beans cooked from scratch, but you can substitute a 14-ounce can of beans as well.

Artichoke Tapenade

SERVES 4

Tangy, lemony, salty, and creamy all at the same time, this sophisticated tapenade is a tasty and healthy alternative to heavier artichoke and spinach dips, and it's much more versatile, too. It's wonderful on crackers if you blend it until chunky, and it's delightful as a dip if you blend it a few more minutes. It will please adults and kids alike.

14 pitted green olives
2 garlic cloves
2 tablespoons fresh parsley, chopped
2 teaspoons capers, drained (optional)
1 tablespoon olive oil
8 to 10 canned artichoke hearts, diced
1 teaspoon freshly squeezed lemon juice
½ teaspoon salt
½ teaspoon freshly ground black pepper

1. In a food processor, blend the olives, garlic, parsley, capers, and oil. Transfer to a small bowl.
2. Add the diced artichokes and mix. Add the lemon juice, salt, and pepper and mix. Cover and refrigerate for 1 hour. Bring to room temperature to serve.

Creamy Artichoke Dip

SERVES 4

What party is complete without a creamy artichoke dip? Vegans can have it all with this simple and incredibly delicious recipe that Denise, the photographer for this book and Mayim's close friend, always offers to bring to parties. It is so close to the "real deal" that you will want to eat the whole casserole by yourself! Denise presents it with crunchy chunks of bread, and no one—vegan or not—can resist it.

2 (15-ounce) cans artichoke hearts
2 (8-ounce) cans diced chili
1 cup vegan mayonnaise
1 cup vegan Parmesan cheese
8 scallions
2 garlic cloves
Salt and freshly ground black pepper

1. Preheat the oven to 375°F. Put all the ingredients except the salt and pepper in a food processor and blend together until smooth. Season to taste.
2. Transfer to a 9 × 13-inch casserole dish and bake, covered, for 10 minutes. Uncover, stir, and bake for another 15 minutes. Serve hot.

Fava Bean Dip

If you've never eaten a fava bean, this recipe will change that for the better. Fava beans have a rich and starchy texture and a flavor that rivals hummus, and serving this dip alongside hummus with freshly cut veggies will have people vying for more. If you buy favas fresh, prepare to spend some time opening the pods, but know that frozen favas work great in this recipe, too. You will be amazed at how you went this long without getting to know and love fava beans.

2½ pounds fava beans in the pod, or 10 ounces frozen
¾ cup olive oil
1 small sprig rosemary
1 garlic clove, minced
¾ teaspoon sea salt
¼ teaspoon freshly ground black pepper
Juice of ½ lemon

1. Preheat the oven to 375°F. Bring a medium pot of salted water to a boil over high heat. Have ready a bowl of ice water.
2. Meanwhile, remove the beans from their pods (or thaw the frozen favas). Blanch the beans for about 2 minutes in the boiling water. Drain the beans in a colander, cool them in the ice water, and then slip them out of their shells with your fingers.
3. Heat a medium saucepan over low heat. Pour in the olive oil and add the rosemary sprig. Let it sizzle in the oil for a minute, then stir in the garlic. Cook for 1 minute and then stir in the fava beans, salt, and pepper. Simmer the beans for 5 to7 minutes, stirring occasionally, until they're tender (the exact time will depend on the starchiness of the favas). Strain out the beans, reserving the oil. Discard the rosemary.
4. Transfer the beans to a food processor. With the motor running, pour in half of the reserved oil slowly, and add more until the puree is velvety smooth. (The amount of oil you will need to add depends on the starchiness of the beans.) Squeeze in some lemon juice and season with salt and pepper to taste.

French Onion Dip

MAKES 1 CUP DIP

This simple recipe Mayim got from her mother combines vegan sour cream and vegan mayonnaise for a traditional party favorite. Serve with fresh vegetables or crackers.

½ cup vegan sour cream
½ cup vegan mayonnaise
3 tablespoons Lipton onion soup mix (see Kitchen Tip)
1 teaspoon dried dill
1 teaspoon onion, minced (optional)

1. Combine all the ingredients in a medium bowl. Chill until ready to serve.

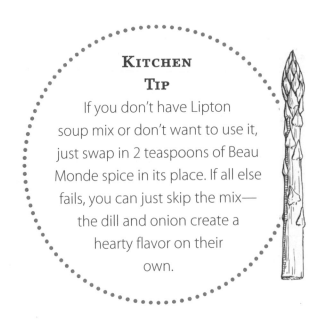

KITCHEN TIP

If you don't have Lipton soup mix or don't want to use it, just swap in 2 teaspoons of Beau Monde spice in its place. If all else fails, you can just skip the mix— the dill and onion create a hearty flavor on their own.

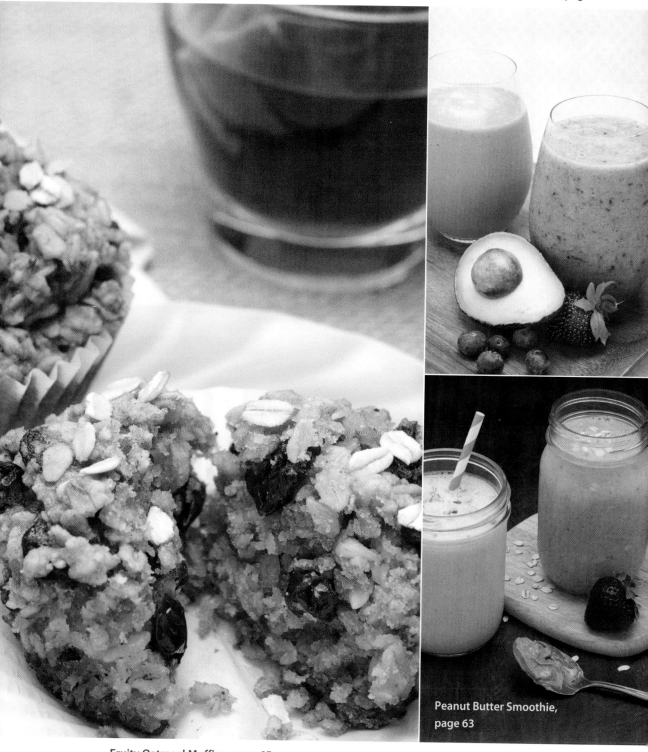

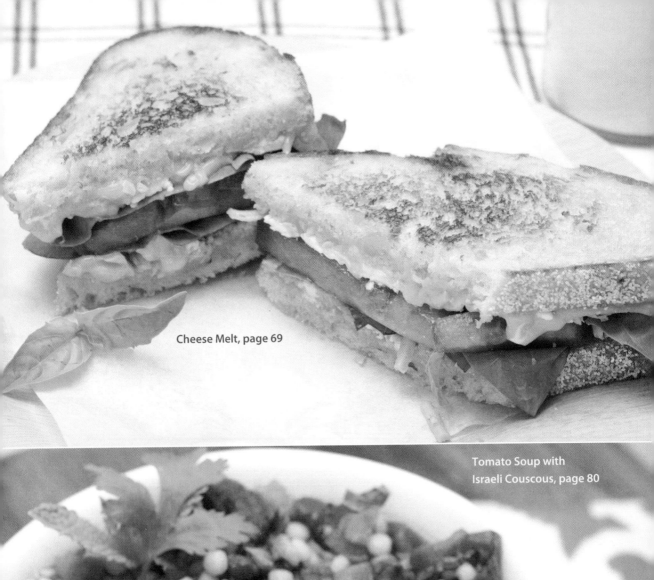

Cheese Melt, page 69

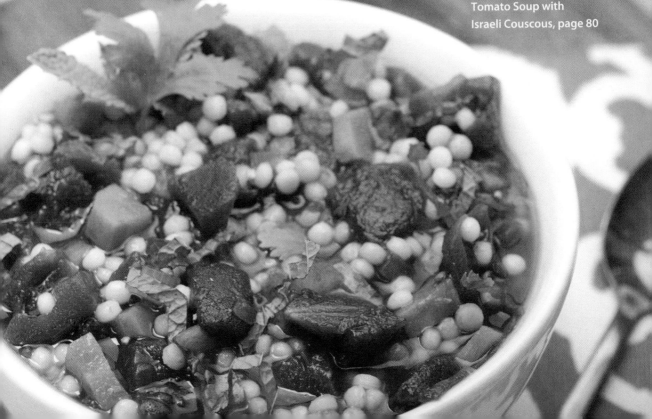

Tomato Soup with
Israeli Couscous, page 80

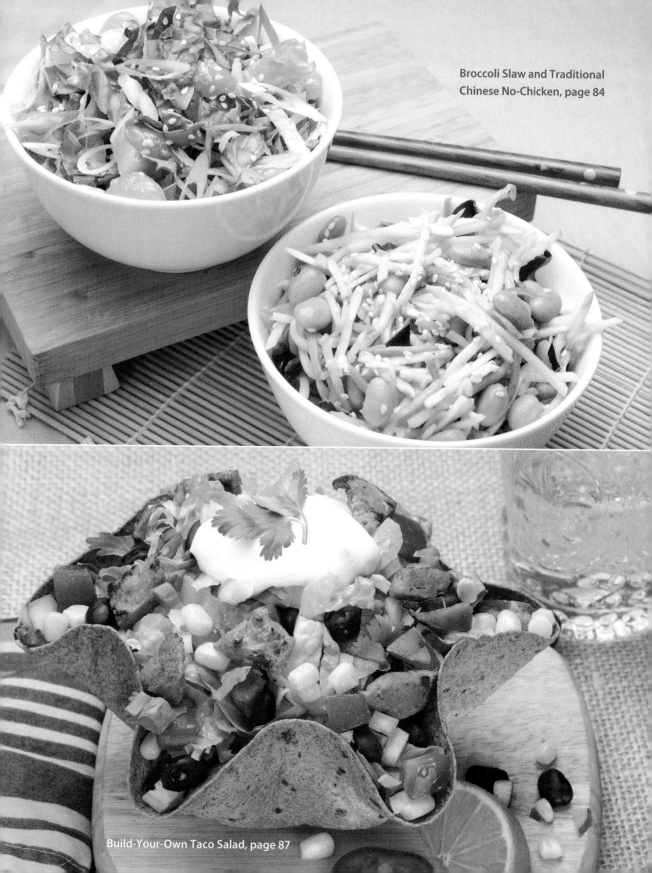

Broccoli Slaw and Traditional Chinese No-Chicken, page 84

Build-Your-Own Taco Salad, page 87

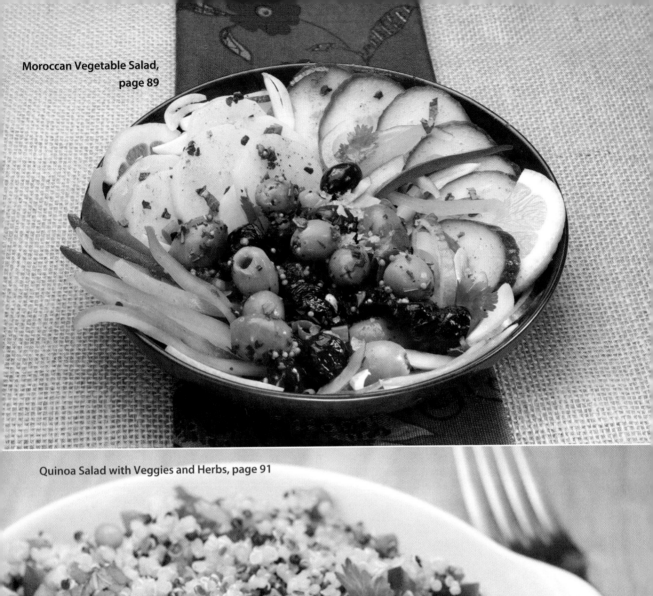

Moroccan Vegetable Salad, page 89

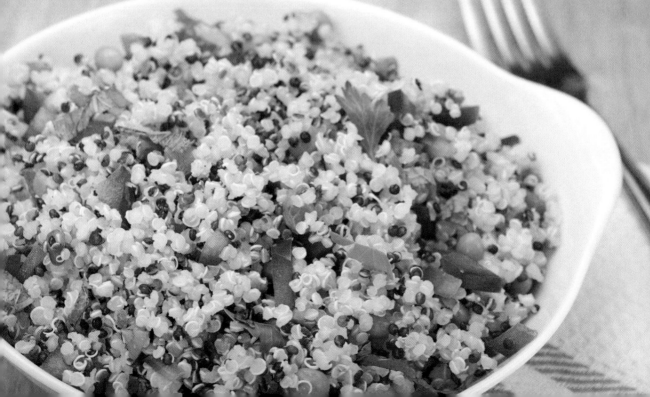

Quinoa Salad with Veggies and Herbs, page 91

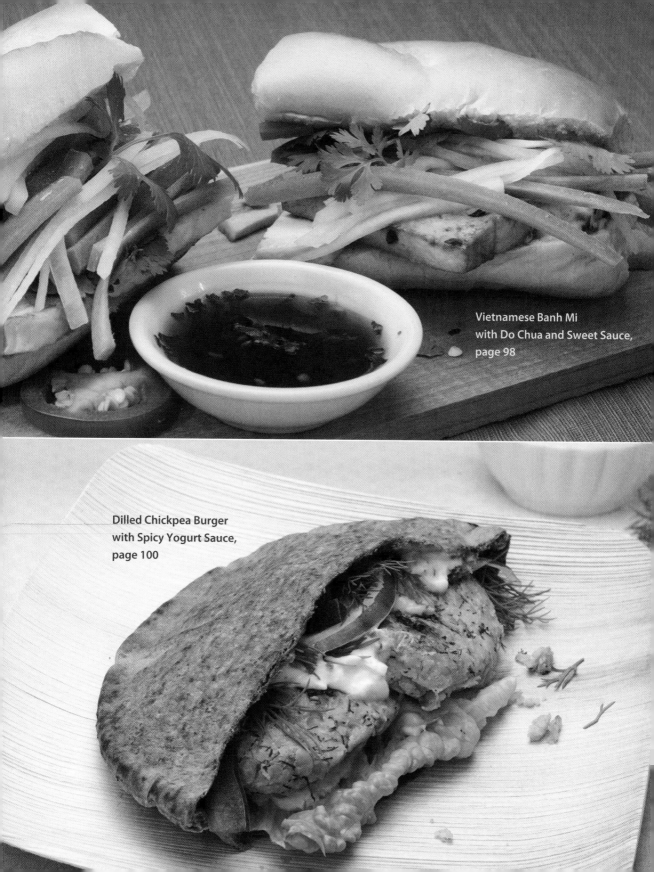

Vietnamese Banh Mi
with Do Chua and Sweet Sauce,
page 98

Dilled Chickpea Burger
with Spicy Yogurt Sauce,
page 100

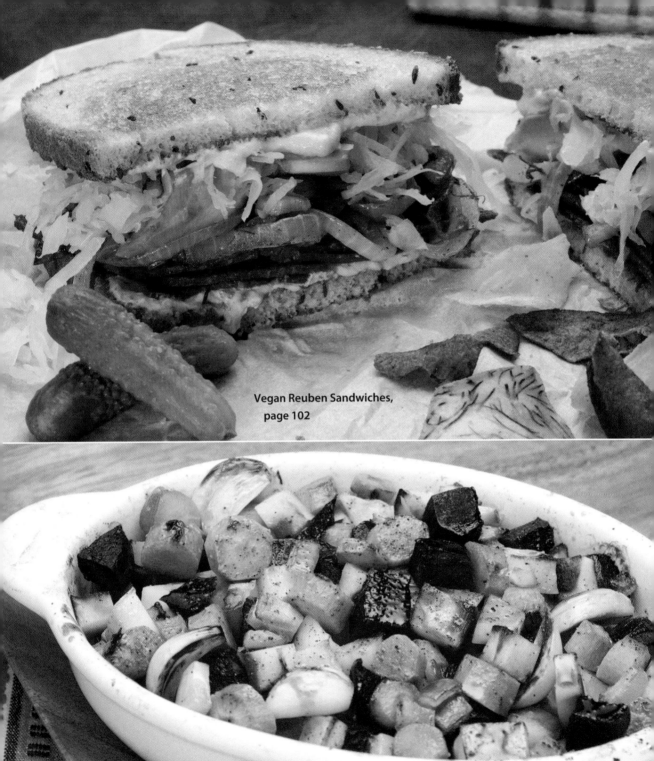

Vegan Reuben Sandwiches,
page 102

Tzimmes, page 125

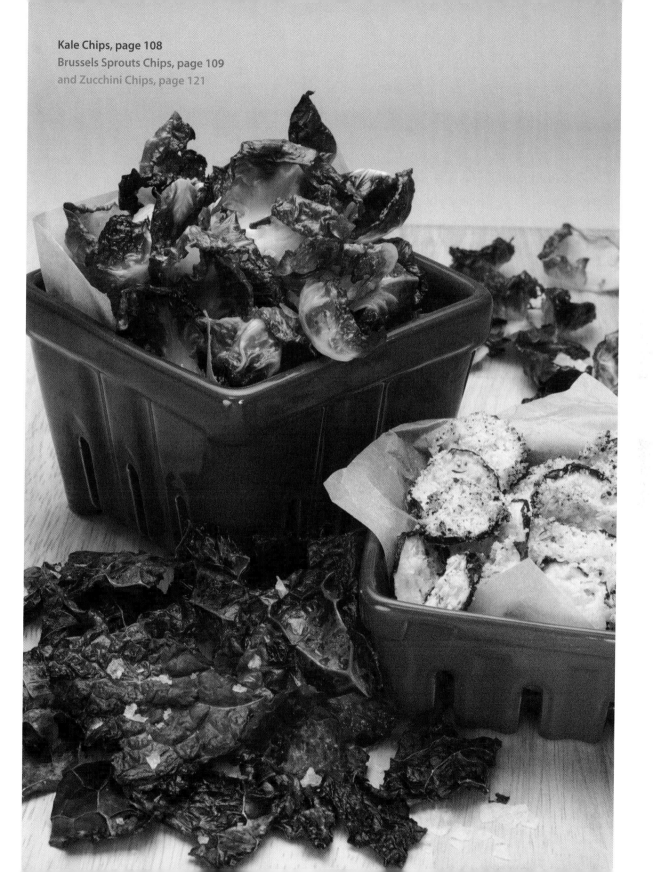

Kale Chips, page 108
Brussels Sprouts Chips, page 109
and Zucchini Chips, page 121

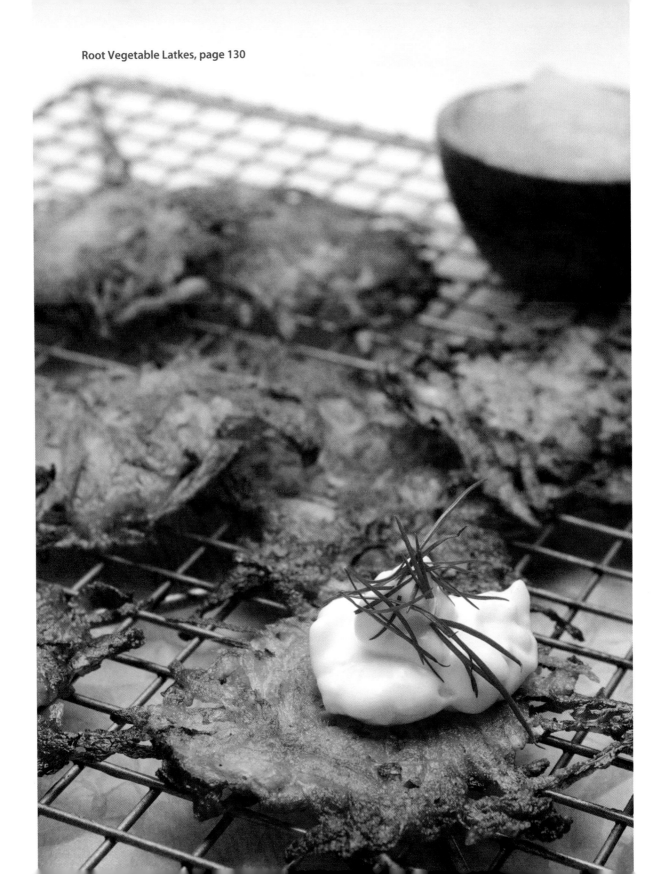

Root Vegetable Latkes, page 130

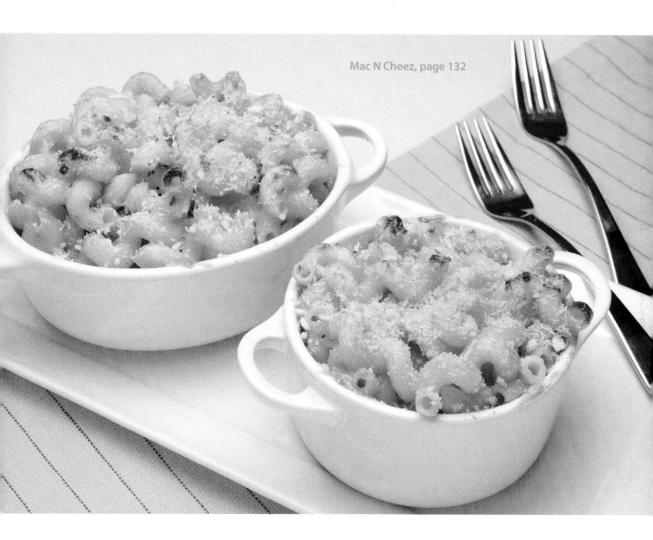
Mac N Cheez, page 132

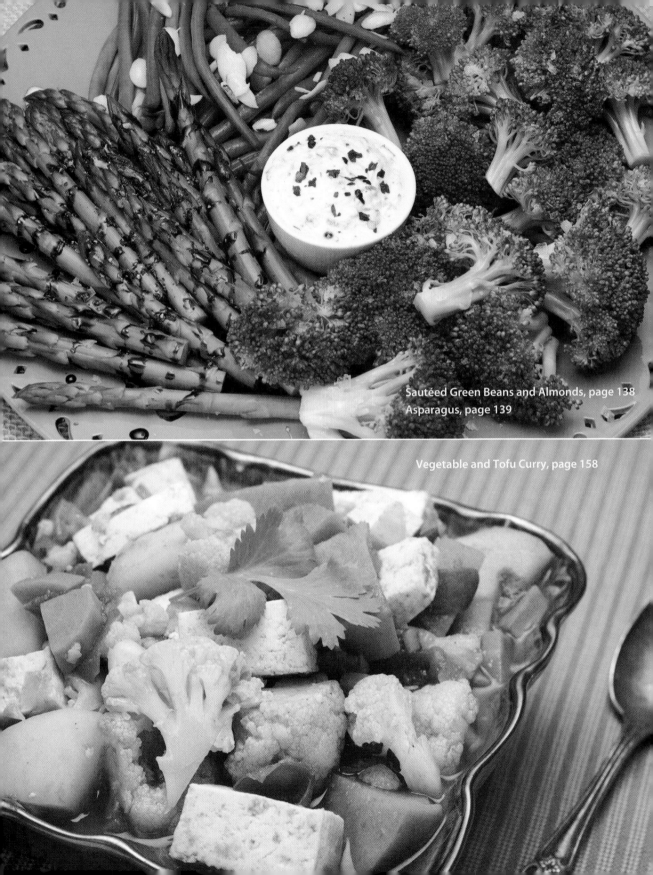

Sautéed Green Beans and Almonds, page 138
Asparagus, page 139

Vegetable and Tofu Curry, page 158

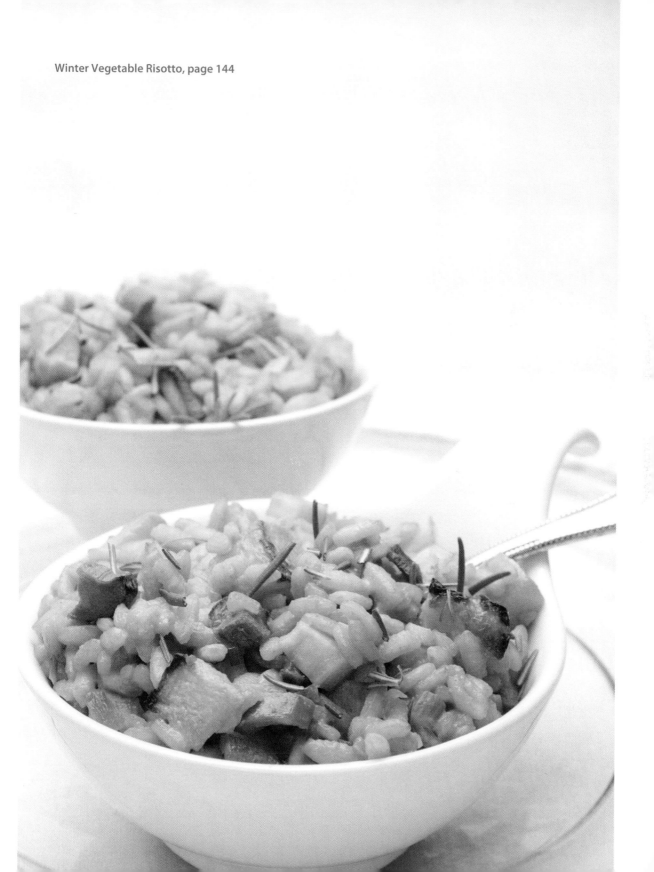

Winter Vegetable Risotto, page 144

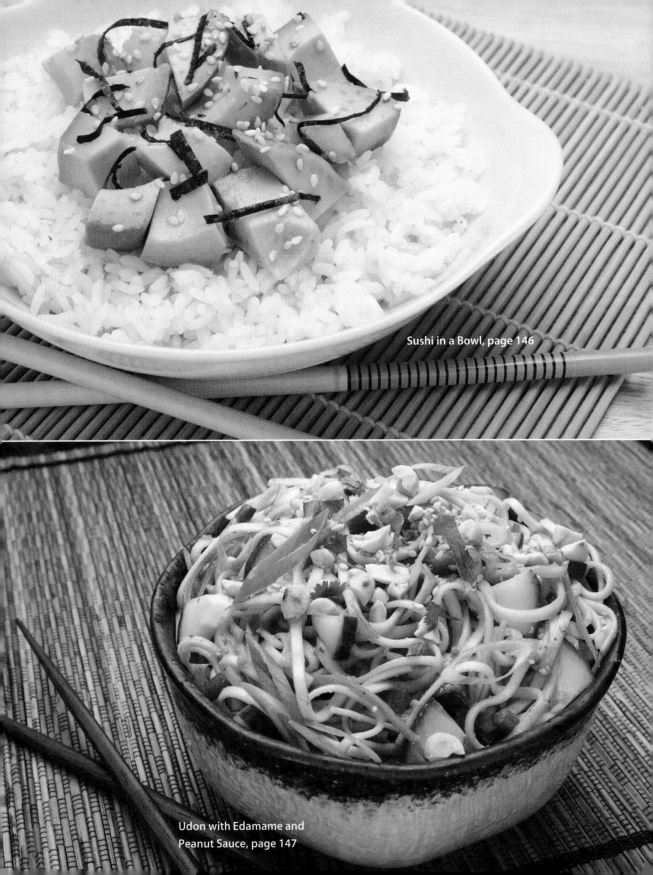

Sushi in a Bowl, page 146

Udon with Edamame and
Peanut Sauce, page 147

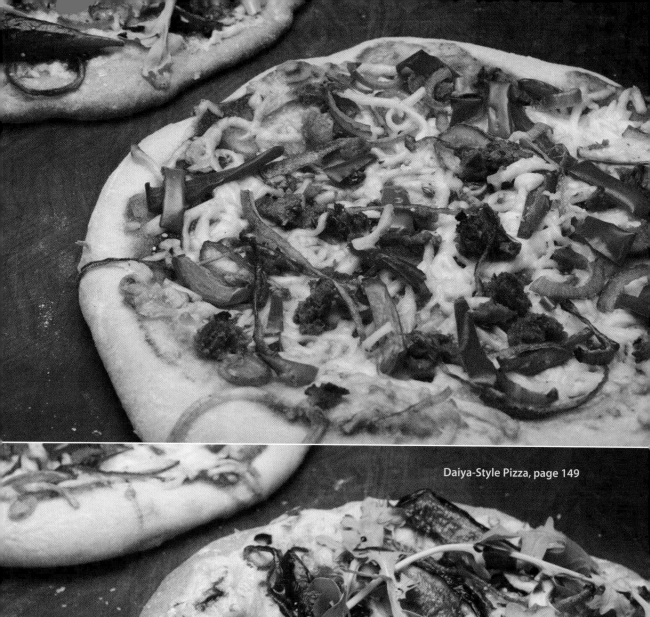
Daiya-Style Pizza, page 149
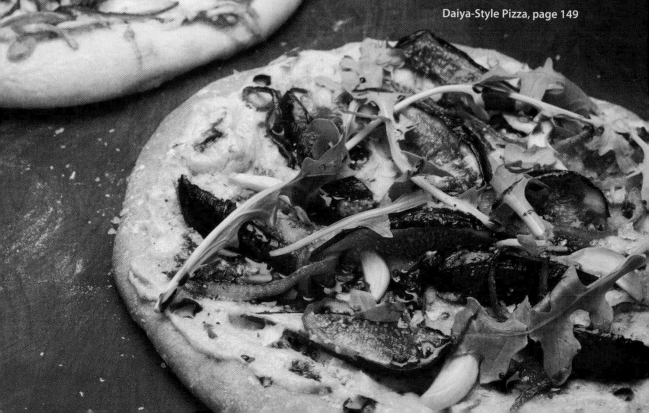

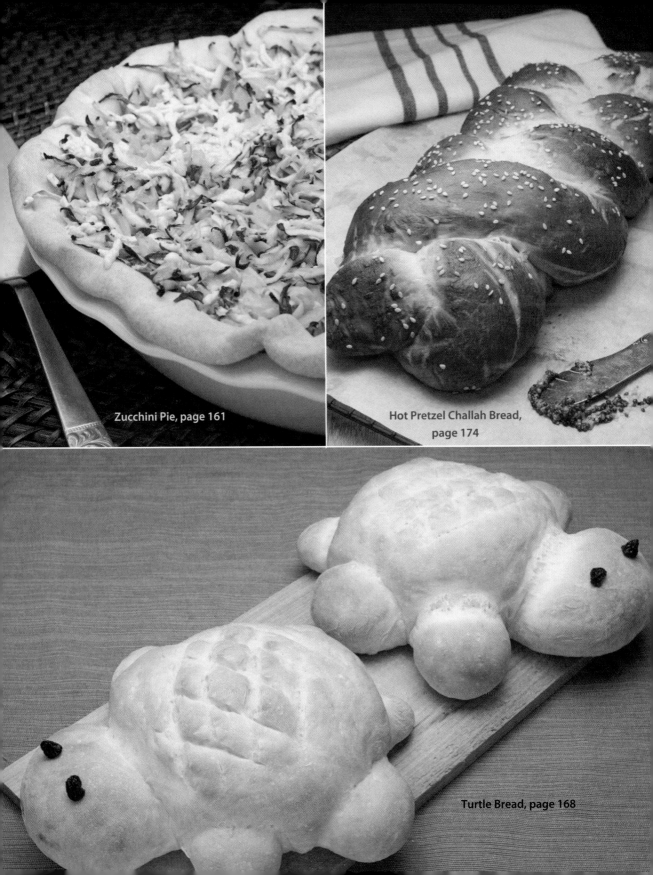

Zucchini Pie, page 161

Hot Pretzel Challah Bread, page 174

Turtle Bread, page 168

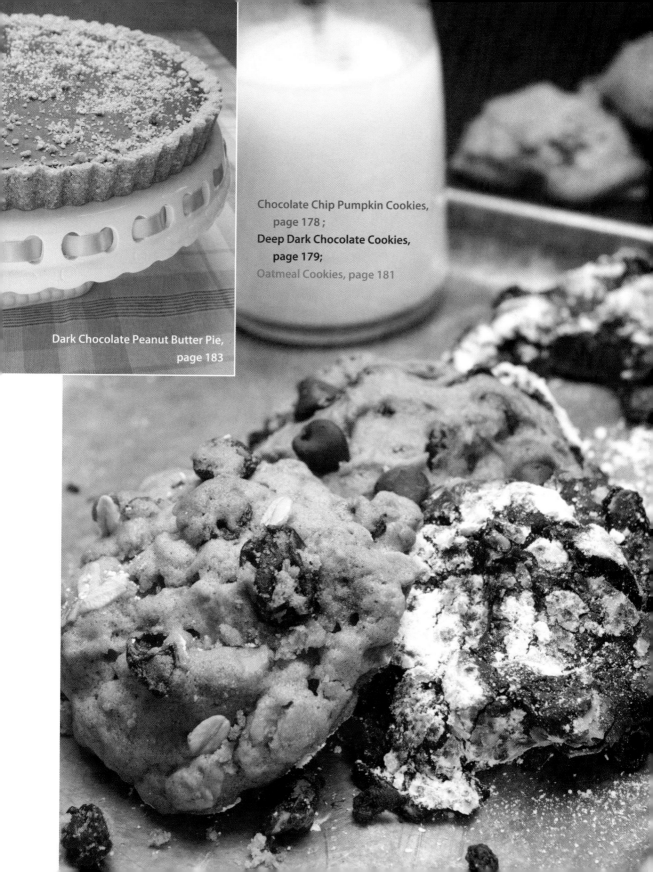

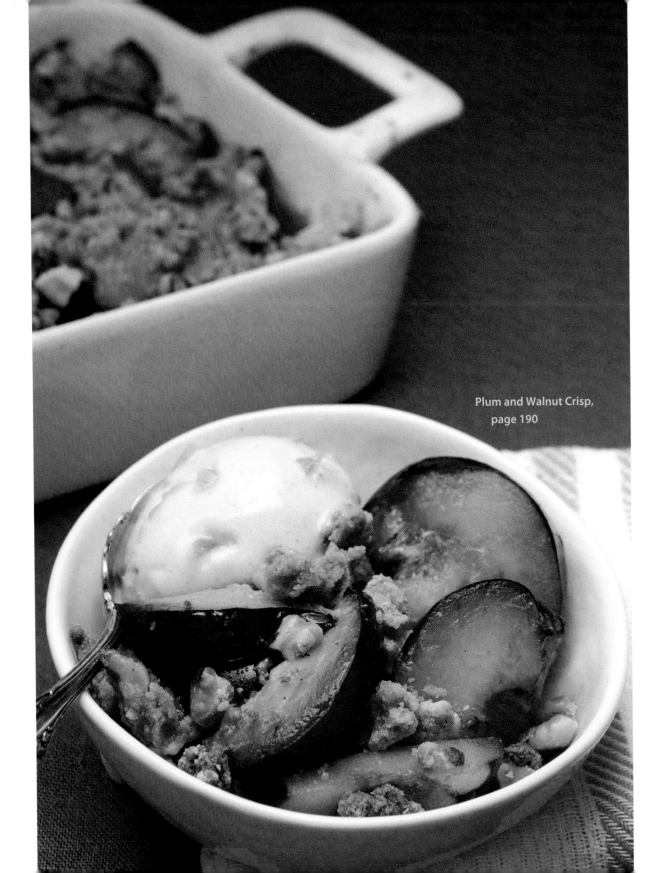

Plum and Walnut Crisp,
page 190

Eggplant and Red Pepper Crostini

SERVES 4

If you've never cooked eggplant, grilling over an open flame is an easy way to take the skin off. Adding red pepper, vinegar, and plenty of garlic makes a colorful, rich and savory Middle Eastern–inspired topping for crostini.

2 eggplants
2 red bell peppers
3 garlic cloves, minced
Juice of ½ lemon
½ teaspoon sherry or wine vinegar
3 tablespoons olive oil

¼ teaspoon coarse sea salt
1 baguette, sliced thinly and toasted

1. Place the eggplants and peppers directly over a medium-low gas flame or over a hot grill. Turn the vegetables frequently until they are evenly charred, 8 to 10 minutes. Put the eggplant and peppers in a bowl and seal tightly. Let cool for 30 to 40 minutes.
2. Peel the vegetables over the bowl, discarding skins and reserving the juices. Roughly chop the vegetables and return them to the bowl. Add the juices, garlic, lemon, vinegar, olive oil, and salt. Mix well to combine. Serve on baguette slices.

Pesto Crostini

SERVES 4

Pesto is typically cheese-based, but this vegan version loses none of the creaminess when it loses the cheese. You can use pine nuts but you can also use just about any nut as a base, and you can also vary the amount of greens and garlic depending on your taste. Don't just use this pesto on crostini: it's delicious on pizzas, pastas, and makes a great dip for vegetables or a spread on crackers.

2 garlic cloves
4 cups spinach
1 cup fresh basil leaves
Juice of ½ lemon
1 cup raw almonds, walnuts, or pine nuts
½ teaspoon sea salt

1 baguette, toasted

1. Chop the garlic in a food processor, add the remaining ingredients, except the bread, and blend well.
2. Serve on toasted baguette slices.

KITCHEN TIP

Softer nuts, such as walnuts and pecans, can be blended nicely in any standard blender or chopper. Harder nuts, such as almonds and cashews, blend most easily in a high-powered blender, such as the ones we discuss in Chapter 4's Gadgets and Things section (page 56).

Bruschetta

SERVES 4

Bruschetta is an Italian toast with a tomato topping. Let the marinade soak into the vegetables for at least a few hours to meld the flavors.

4 medium-size tomatoes, diced
1 red onion, diced
¼ cup olive oil
2 tablespoons balsamic vinegar
2 garlic cloves, minced
1 teaspoon sea salt
¼ teaspoon freshly ground black pepper

8 slices thick crusty bread, toasted

1. Place the diced vegetables in a bowl. Drizzle with the olive oil and vinegar. Add the garlic, salt, and pepper, and stir to combine. Cover and refrigerate at least 1 hour. Spread onto toasted bread.

Hummus

SERVES 4

It seems everyone loves hummus for its simple ingredients, high protein content, and its flexibility as a dip or spread. Here's Dr. Jay's favorite recipe for do-it-yourself hummus. Add chopped olives, sun-dried tomatoes, or basil to give the hummus extra kick, if desired.

2 (14-ounce) cans chickpeas, drained and rinsed
½ teaspoon garlic, minced
1½ teaspoons salt
5 tablespoons freshly squeezed lemon juice
⅓ cup tahini
¼ cup olive oil

1. In a food processor, combine the chickpeas, garlic, and salt. Puree for about 30 seconds. Scrape down the sides of the bowl and puree for another 30 seconds. Add the lemon juice and ¼ cup of water and puree for another 30 seconds. Add the tahini and puree for 30 more seconds. Scrape down the sides of the bowl. With the processor running, drizzle in the olive oil. Mix until well blended.

Zucchini Chips

SERVES 4

These zucchini chips are a healthy alternative to fried appetizers, as they are breaded and baked. Excellent for dipping and wonderful for little hands to help assemble, eat these straight from the oven for optimal crispiness.

½ cup bread crumbs

¼ cup vegan Parmesan cheese (optional)

½ teaspoon salt

¼ teaspoon freshly ground black pepper

½ teaspoon garlic powder

1 teaspoon dried Italian seasoning

1 cup plain, unsweetened soy or rice milk

4 medium-size zucchini, cut into ¼-inch-thick coins

1. Preheat the oven to 425°F. In a shallow bowl, mix together the bread crumbs, vegan cheese (if using), spices, and herbs.
2. Pour the nondairy milk into a small bowl. Dip the zucchini slices into the milk and then into the bread crumb mixture. Place each slice on a baking rack placed on a sheet pan and bake for 30 minutes.
3. Remove from the oven and serve hot.

CHAPTER 8

Veggies and Sides

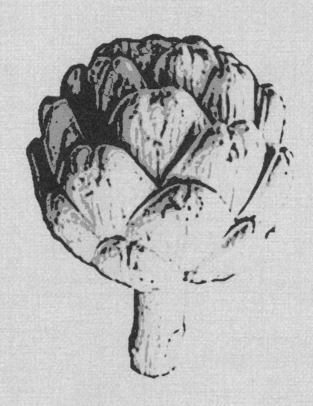

Agaved Carrots

Honeyed carrots is a standard recipe for the Jewish New Year. The round shapes and the sweetness echo the cycle of the year and hopes for sweet things to come. This vegan version tastes just like the honeyed version. It makes a sweet side dish to complement a fall-themed menu or any hearty meal that merits a creative and colorful vegetable side dish.

1 pound carrots
2 tablespoons vegetable oil
3 tablespoons agave nectar
Juice of 2 oranges
½ teaspoon salt
Handful of raisins

1. Slice the carrots thinly. Pour the vegetable oil into the bottom of a medium saucepan. Put in the carrots first, then the other ingredients. Cover and simmer for about 30 minutes over low heat, checking occasionally to make sure the carrots don't burn. Serve hot.

Tzimmes

SERVES 4

Eastern European Jews will recognize this dish as a motley assembly of root vegetables and onions with a sweet, light marinade. The Yiddish word means "a fuss." Tzimmes is tastiest when the vegetables get a tad mushed together. It is a wonderful side dish at any meal where you have to please a lot of mouths, as the ingredients are not expensive. The final result is hearty and satisfying, and the sweet and rich taste is a sure hit.

4 large carrots, diced
2 beets, peeled and diced
1 large red onion, diced
1 large sweet potato, diced
6 garlic cloves, unpeeled
3 tablespoons olive oil
3 tablespoons balsamic vinegar
1 tablespoon soy sauce
1 tablespoon agave nectar
1 tablespoon paprika
2 teaspoons salt
½ teaspoon freshly ground black pepper
Juice of 1 orange

1. Preheat the oven to 350°F. Place the vegetables in an 8-inch glass baking dish. Arrange the garlic cloves around the veggies. Drizzle with the olive oil, vinegar, soy sauce, and agave nectar and sprinkle with the paprika, sea salt, and pepper. Squeeze the orange juice over the whole thing, cover, and bake for 45 minutes, until tender.

Golden Couscous
with Olives and Fresh Herbs

SERVES 8

Mayim likes to make this dish for festive meals, such as on Shabbat, when special dishes are paraded. The dish calls for the larger Israeli couscous, and it has a rich flavor and a beautiful gold color, thanks to the turmeric. You can add other vegetables to make it more substantial, or leave it as is for a side dish. Substitute quinoa for the couscous for more protein and a slightly lighter version.

8 tablespoons (1 stick) vegan margarine

6 cups onion, chopped

¾ teaspoon ground ginger

½ teaspoon turmeric

2¼ cups low-salt vegan chicken-flavored stock

1 cup pitted and halved kalamata olives

½ cup fresh basil, chopped

⅓ cup fresh mint, chopped

¼ cup freshly squeezed lemon juice

2 cups uncooked Israeli couscous

Salt and freshly ground black pepper

1. Melt the margarine in a large, heavy-bottomed pot over medium-low heat. Add the onion and stir to coat. Cover and sauté until the onion is very tender but not browned, stirring occasionally, about 10 minutes. Mix in the ginger and turmeric. Add the stock, olives, basil, mint, and lemon juice and bring to simmer. Stir in the couscous. Cover the pot, turn off the heat, and let stand until all liquid is absorbed and the couscous is tender, about 10 minutes.
2. Fluff the couscous with a fork. Season to taste with salt and pepper.

Spanish Rice

SERVES 4

While brown rice is a staple in many vegan homes, this Spanish variation is fun with burritos or tacos, or even sprinkled over a taco salad for extra flavor. This simple dish has that authentic flavor you get in a restaurant, and if you serve it with grilled or sautéed vegetables, it makes a satisfying complete meal.

3 tablespoons vegetable oil
1 cup uncooked long-grain rice
1 teaspoon garlic salt
½ teaspoon ground cumin
¼ cup onion, chopped
½ cup tomato sauce
2 cups vegan chicken-flavored stock

1. Heat the oil in a large saucepan over medium heat and add the rice. Cook, stirring constantly, until the rice is puffed and golden, about 4 minutes. While the rice is cooking, sprinkle with the garlic salt and cumin.
2. Stir in the onion and cook until tender. Stir in the tomato sauce and stock and bring to a boil. Lower the heat to low, cover, and simmer for 20 to 25 minutes. Fluff with a fork.

Corn Bread Thanksgiving Dressing

SERVES 8

Mayim's sons' great-grandmother is from Louisiana, and this corn bread recipe is a classic in her family. Her recipe was scrawled on a note card and called for "a few plump chickens," "lots of eggs," and "2 large jars of mayonnaise." We veganized it and toned down the fat content, but everyone who has had both this version and the "original" says they are almost indistinguishable! This soupy mixture of onions, corn bread, croutons, apples, and celery gets its flavor from a vegan stock and vegan mayonnaise, but it bakes into an incredibly rich and satisfying stuffing. It keeps well for days and days, so make enough for leftovers. You'll be glad you did.

1 (20-ounce) package vegan cornbread mix, prepared;
   or 1 recipe CREAMED CORN BREAD, PAGE 166
1 (16-ounce) package seasoned bread crumbs
2 large white onions, chopped
4 large red apples, cored and finely chopped
64 ounces vegan vegetable or chicken-flavored stock
1 cup vegan mayonnaise
5 celery stalks, diced

1. Preheat the oven to 350°F. Mix all the ingredients together in a large roaster pan or a 9 × 13-inch baking dish. It will be soupy. Bake for an hour, or until starting to brown.

Latkes

SERVES 4

Potato pancakes, or latkes *as they are called in Yiddish, are a classic treat served with applesauce and sour cream for Chanukah. On Chanukah, foods fried in oil recall the historical significance of the miracle of oil, which occurred over two thousand years ago. This veganized version uses egg replacer as a binder, but you can't tell the difference. When fried to a crisp brown and served with applesauce or vegan sour cream, they are the authentic latke experience. When topped with ketchup, they will taste like the best hash browns ever. Drain them well before serving so they are not greasy, but don't skimp on the oil when frying; the best latkes need to be saturated with oil to come out right!*

4 russet or golden potatoes

1 onion

¼ cup matzoh meal, or all-purpose flour if matzoh meal isn't available (Mayim thinks matzoh meal works better!)

Egg replacer equivalent of 1 egg

Pinch of baking soda

1 teaspoon salt

¼ teaspoon freshly ground black pepper

1 cup vegetable oil, for frying

1. Shred the potatoes and onion and place in a strainer over a large bowl. Drain for about 15 minutes, and then discard any liquid in the bowl, leaving any remaining starch. Place the shredded potato and onion mixture and the remaining ingredients in the bowl, and mix well.

2. Heat the oil in a large skillet until very hot but not smoking. Scoop up handful-size patties and place in the hot oil, spreading them into 3- to 4-inch rounds with a fork. You may need to do this in several batches to avoid overcrowding the pan. Don't flip them too much! Fry until golden, about 4 minutes on each side, and drain on paper towels or brown paper bags on a wire rack.

Root Vegetable Latkes

SERVES 4

This colorful vegetable-infused version of classic latkes almost makes up for the fact that they are fried. We serve these with salad and soup, so that the fried food does not become the main event. Serve with ketchup or vegan sour cream, or eat them plain, as they are sweeter than classic latkes, due to the carrots and yams. Drain well before serving so they don't get greasy.

2 russet potatoes

2 carrots

1 sweet potato

1 zucchini

1 red onion

1 bunch fresh dill, minced

2 scallions, sliced

¼ cup matzoh meal or all-purpose flour (see previous recipe)

Egg replacer equivalent of 1 egg

Pinch of baking soda

1 teaspoon salt

½ teaspoon freshly ground black pepper

1 cup vegetable oil, for frying

1. Shred the potatoes, vegetables, and red onion and place in a strainer over a large bowl. Drain for about 15 minutes, and then discard any liquid in the bowl, leaving any remaining starch. Add the shredded vegetables and the remaining ingredients to the bowl, and mix well.

2. Heat the oil in a large skillet until very hot but not smoking. Scoop up handful-size patties and place in the hot oil, spreading them into 3- to 4-inch rounds with a fork. You may need to do this in batches to avoid overcrowding the pan. Don't flip them too much! Fry until golden, about 4 minutes on each side, and drain on paper towels or brown paper bags on a wire rack.

Nondairy Kugel

SERVES 8

Kugel is a popular casserole in Eastern European Jewish homes, and comes in many varieties. This vegan version of a dairy kugel is cheesy and rich. It tastes a bit like macaroni and cheese—in fact, this is quite similar, but with a touch of sour cream for that classic and slightly tart kugel taste. Serve as a side dish or eat as a main course.

1 (16-ounce) package pasta, such as farfalle, shells, or large macaroni
½ onion, diced (optional)
1¼ cups nondairy milk (almond milk works well)
2 tablespoons all-purpose flour or white or brown rice flour
1 (8-ounce) package shredded vegan cheese, preferably mozzarella or cheddar
3 tablespoons vegan margarine
3 tablespoons vegan sour cream
½ cup bread crumbs (optional)

1. Cook the pasta according to the package directions. When al dente, drain and place in a large bowl.
2. Preheat the oven to 350°F. Mix the onion, if desired, with the cooked pasta.
3. Heat 1 cup of the nondairy milk in a medium saucepan over medium heat.
4. In a cup, whisk the flour into the remaining ¼ cup of milk until dissolved. Add it slowly to the heated milk, whisking as you go. Add the shredded vegan cheese and stir constantly until the cheese dissolves and the sauce is bubbly, about 5 minutes. Add the margarine and vegan sour cream to the sauce and stir to combine. Pour over the pasta mixture and mix well.
5. Place in a 9 × 13-inch casserole dish and cover with the bread crumbs. Bake, covered, for 20 minutes, until heated through. Uncover and broil until browned on top, about 5 minutes.

Mac N Cheez

SERVES 8

People often ask vegan children if they miss macaroni and cheese. With this recipe, your kids don't have to miss out on the creamy comfort food many kids think comes from a box. The vegan cheese sauce can be poured and mixed directly into cooked pasta or baked in a casserole. Either way, it is an exceptionally yummy and satisfying dish you'll find yourself making when you crave comfort food in a jiffy.

1 (16-ounce) package pasta, such as farfalle, rigatoni, penne, shells, or large macaroni
1¼ cups nondairy milk (almond milk works best)
2 tablespoons all-purpose flour or white or brown rice flour
1 (8-ounce) bag shredded vegan cheese, preferably mozzarella or cheddar
½ cup bread crumbs (optional)

1. Cook the pasta according to the package directions. Drain when al dente and place in a large bowl.
2. Preheat the oven to 350°F.
3. Heat 1 cup of the nondairy milk in a medium saucepan over medium heat.
4. In a cup, whisk the flour into the remaining ¼ cup of milk until dissolved. Add it slowly to the heated milk, whisking as you go. Add the shredded vegan cheese and stir constantly until the cheese is dissolved and the sauce is bubbly, about 5 minutes. Pour over the pasta mixture and stir to combine.

Sprout and Potato Croquettes
with Dipping Sauce

SERVES 8

Brussels sprouts are such a neglected vegetable! We couldn't resist pairing the sprouts with mashed potato and frying them into a fun shape. These croquettes make a neat side dish, or you can serve them with a nutritious soup or salad to balance out the fun factor of frying. Make sure to drain the croquettes well before serving.

8 ounces brussels sprouts

1 pound potatoes, cooked and mashed

Salt and freshly ground black pepper

¼ cup all-purpose flour

Egg replacer equivalent of 1 egg

½ cup vegan seasoned bread crumbs

1¼ cups vegetable oil, for frying

DIPPING SAUCE

1 (14-ounce) can tomatoes, chopped

¼ cup fresh cilantro, chopped

1 teaspoon vegetarian Worcestershire sauce

1 shallot, finely sliced

1. Drop the sprouts into boiling water and blanch for 2 to 3 minutes. Drain and refresh with cold water. Combine with the mashed potato, mashing them together with a fork. Season well and form into twelve cylinder-shaped croquettes.

2. Place the flour on a plate, the egg replacer in a bowl, and the bread crumbs on a second plate.

3. Dip each croquette into the flour first, to coat, then into the egg, and lastly, into the bread crumbs. Make sure each is fully covered. Chill in the fridge for 30 minutes, or up to 24 hours.

4. To make the dip, combine all the ingredients in a small bowl.

5. Pour the oil into a large, deep skillet, to a depth of about 1½ inches, and place over medium-high heat. Fry the croquettes until golden, a total of 5 minutes. You may need to do this in two batches to avoid overcrowding the pan. Drain on paper towels and serve immediately.

Spice-Crusted Baby Potatoes
with Tamarind Cream

SERVES 8

So many roasted potato recipes call for simply herbs and olive oil, but in our opinion, this potato recipe packs much more flavor and class. Tiny potatoes are coated with zesty herbs, with a bright tamarind cream dipping sauce on the side. They make a great appetizer or side dish. Way to class up potatoes!

1 teaspoon ground coriander

1 teaspoon ground cumin

½ teaspoon turmeric

½ teaspoon cayenne pepper

1 teaspoon salt

3 tablespoons olive oil

1 tablespoon red wine vinegar

2 pounds baby potatoes

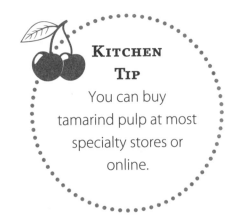

KITCHEN TIP

You can buy tamarind pulp at most specialty stores or online.

TAMARIND CREAM

½ cup vegan sour cream

½ cup soy yogurt

2 tablespoons tamarind pulp (see Kitchen Tip)

1. Preheat the oven to 350°F. In a small bowl, whisk the spices with the oil and vinegar. Place the potatoes in a 9 × 13-inch baking dish and pour in the spice mixture. Cover the dish with aluminum foil and bake for 35 to 45 minutes, until the potatoes are tender and can be pierced easily with a fork. Transfer the potatoes to a serving dish and set the leftover spices aside to use in the dipping sauce.

2. To make the tamarind cream, mix all the ingredients in a medium-size bowl, adding the remaining spice mixture from the potatoes. Serve on the side as a dipping sauce.

Oven-Baked Fries

SERVES 4

Mayim's mom has been making oven-baked french fries since Mayim was a kid. Mayim resented her for it then, but now sees the value and enthusiastically supports oven-baked fries. If they're baked long enough to be crispy, kids won't be able to tell the difference. And with a few fun dips, such as vegan ranch dressing, ketchup, or agave nectar mixed with mustard, these will disappear in a flash.

4 medium-size russet or sweet potatoes
3 tablespoons vegetable oil
Salt

1. Preheat the oven to at 350°F. Cut the potatoes lengthwise into thick wedges. Halve, quarter, and then quarter again to make eight spears.
2. In a large bowl, toss the potatoes and vegetable oil, then arrange in a single layer on a rimmed baking sheet. Sprinkle with salt and bake for 25 minutes, until starting to brown.

Oven-Baked Parsnip Fries

SERVES 4

Here's an unusual take on the oven-baked french fry, which is equally delicious and just as easy to make. Parsnips are like a jazzed-up potato. They provide great flavor and a beautiful appearance.

2 pounds parsnips
¼ cup grapeseed oil
1 teaspoon salt
½ teaspoon freshly ground black pepper

1. Preheat the oven to 350°F. Remove the tops from the parsnips, then peel and slice into French fry–like strips. Place the oil, salt, and pepper in a medium-size bowl. Add the parsnips and toss to coat.
2. Arrange the parsnips in a single layer on a rimmed baking sheet, and bake for 25 minutes, until crisp and starting to brown.

Maple Mustard Greens

SERVES 4

How do you get kids to eat dark greens? This recipe. Greens like these are high in so many nutrients, including vitamins K, A, and C, folate, and calcium. A little maple syrup makes them sweet without losing their nutritional value.

1 bunch Swiss or rainbow chard
1 bunch kale
1 bunch collard greens
¼ cup Dijon mustard
¼ cup whole-grain mustard
¼ cup maple syrup
1 teaspoon salt
½ teaspoon freshly ground black pepper
1 tablespoon olive oil, for frying

1. Clean and dry all the greens. Tear the leaves off the stems into medium-size pieces and place in a large bowl.
2. Mix the mustards and maple syrup in a small bowl. Pour over the greens and toss to coat. Add the salt and pepper.
3. Heat the oil in a large skillet over high heat. Add the greens and sauté just until wilted, about 5 minutes. Serve immediately.

Sautéed Green Beans and Almonds

SERVES 4

Green beans get a makeover in this side dish, with a simple lemon-butter vinaigrette and slivered almonds for crunch and protein. This dish is yummy served warm or cold.

1 pound green beans, trimmed
2 tablespoons slivered almonds
2 tablespoons vegan margarine
1 teaspoon freshly squeezed lemon juice

1. Bring 8 cups of water and 2 tablespoons of salt to boil in a medium pot. Add the beans and cook until crisp-tender, about 4 minutes.
2. Drain and spoon the beans into a serving bowl.
3. In a small pan over low heat, melt the vegan margarine. Add the almonds and sauté, stirring occasionally, until golden. Watch them as they can burn really quickly. Add to the beans.
4. Pour the melted margarine and lemon juice over the bean mixture.

Asparagus

People know they should eat asparagus but often they don't know how to prepare it. Here's a super simple recipe that lets the asparagus speak for itself. It's important to not let the asparagus get soggy, so watch it closely. You can also lay the asparagus spears on a barbecue grill and grill them over direct heat until bright green but not soggy, about 5 minutes.

1 bunch asparagus, stems trimmed
2 tablespoons olive oil
2 tablespoons balsamic vinegar
Salt and freshly ground black pepper

1. Preheat the oven to 350°F. In a large bowl, toss the asparagus in the oil and vinegar to coat.
2. Transfer to a baking dish and sprinkle with salt and pepper to taste. Roast for 8 to 10 minutes.

Teriyaki Tofu

This tofu dish is a smart choice if you are cooking for people who have never had tofu before, as well as experienced tofu eaters. It uses a basic teriyaki sauce to highlight this popular protein, which is an important part of the vegan diet. You can also marinate the tofu in a good store-bought sauce, such as Soy Vay.

½ cup soy sauce
½ cup mirin
2 tablespoons maple syrup
1 (14-ounce) package extra-firm sprouted tofu
1 tablespoon toasted sesame seeds

1. In a large bowl, mix soy sauce, mirin, and maple syrup together.
2. Remove the sprouted tofu from its container. Wrap it in paper towels and place on a plate for 5 minutes, then cut into ¼-inch-thick slices. Add to the bowl of sauce and let marinate for about 2 hours in the fridge. You don't need to leave it that long, but the sprouted tofu absorbs more flavor the longer it sits.
3. You can sauté the marinated tofu in a nonstick skillet for 4 to 5 minutes per side. Alternatively, you can bake it on a nonstick baking sheet in a preheated 400°F oven for 15 to 20 minutes, until starting to crisp.
4. On a rimmed baking sheet, toast the seeds for 8 to 10 minutes, watching closely. You can also use a toaster oven until the seeds start to darken, or sauté them without oil in a small pan until they brown and become fragrant, about 5 minutes. Remove from the heat and set aside. Sprinkle over the tofu before serving.

CHAPTER 9

Entrées

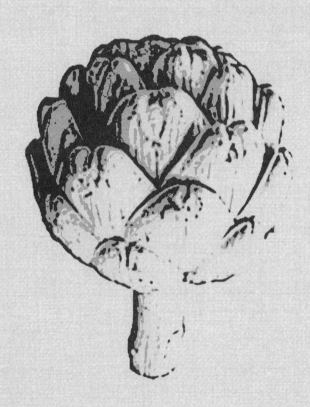

Baked Ziti

SERVES 8

This is the dish Mayim makes for nonvegans that they consistently can't believe is vegan. Pureed tofu and cashew cream mimic mozzarella and ricotta cheese. Whether you make this sauce or substitute a jarred one, the flavors of this ziti are unbelievable. This dish keeps well, so prepare for days of delicious leftovers.

1 tablespoon salt
12 ounces ziti pasta (or penne)
3 tablespoons fresh basil or parsley, chopped, for garnish

HERBED "RICOTTA"
1½ cups raw macadamia nuts, soaked in a bowl of water for at least 4 hours
⅛ teaspoon garlic, minced
½ teaspoon salt
1 tablespoon olive oil

TOMATO SAUCE (OR USE A JAR OF PREPARED VEGAN SAUCE)
1 tablespoon olive oil
½ cup onion, chopped
1 teaspoon garlic, minced
3 teaspoons dried Italian seasoning
1 (14-ounce) can roasted tomatoes, diced
1 (14-ounce) can tomato sauce
1 teaspoon salt

CASHEW CREAM
1 cup raw cashews, soaked for at least 2 hours
½ teaspoon dried oregano
1 teaspoon salt
2 teaspoon freshly squeezed lemon juice
¼ teaspoon rice vinegar
2 tablespoons chopped fresh parsley

1. Bring a pot of salted water to boil and cook the pasta according to the package instructions. Drain and rinse, let cool, and set aside.

2. To make the herbed "ricotta," combine the macadamia nuts, ¼ cup of water, and the garlic, salt, and olive oil in a food processor and puree for 1 minute. Scrape down the sides and puree for another minute, until light and fluffy. Set aside.

3. To make the tomato sauce, heat the olive oil in a medium skillet over high heat, and sauté the onion until soft and translucent, about 8 minutes. Add the garlic and herbs and sauté for another 2 minutes. Lower the heat to medium, add the tomatoes and tomato sauce, and simmer for 30 minutes. Add the salt and cook for another 15 minutes.

4. To make the cashew cream, puree the soaked cashews in a blender until a smooth paste forms. Add ⅓ cup of water and the remaining ingredients and puree until creamy.

5. Preheat the oven to 350°F. To assemble the baked ziti, toss the pasta with the tomato sauce in a large bowl, and then stir in the herbed "ricotta." Mix in the cashew cream.

6. Spread into a 9 × 13-inch baking dish, cover with aluminum foil, and bake for 30 minutes, or until the cheese starts to brown. Garnish with fresh basil or parsley, as desired.

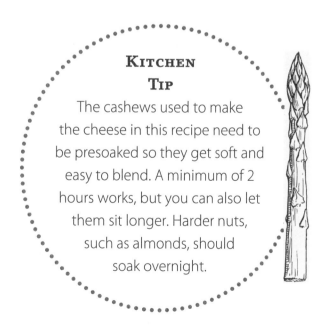

KITCHEN TIP

The cashews used to make the cheese in this recipe need to be presoaked so they get soft and easy to blend. A minimum of 2 hours works, but you can also let them sit longer. Harder nuts, such as almonds, should soak overnight.

Winter Vegetable Risotto

Risotto is often hard to mimic as a vegan dish because it calls for lots of Parmesan and butter to create its creamy taste and consistency. This recipe re-creates all of that, using a combination of almond milk, tahini, and a touch of nutritional yeast. The result is a sophisticated risotto, which we pair with carrots, parsnips, and butternut squash. You can use any vegetables on hand, though, including diced asparagus, zucchini, or other squash.

1 medium-size carrot, peeled and diced

1 medium-size parsnip, peeled and diced

1 (1-pound) butternut squash, peeled, seeded, and diced (about 2 cups)

1 tablespoon fresh rosemary or thyme, chopped

5 tablespoons olive oil

5½ cups vegan vegetable stock

½ cup dry white wine

2 garlic cloves, minced

1 cup onion or shallot, chopped

1½ cups uncooked arborio rice

½ cup plain, unsweetened almond milk (rice or soy milk works, too)

2 tablespoons tahini

¼ cup nutritional yeast

1 tablespoon freshly squeezed lemon juice

1 tablespoon mirin (see Kitchen Tip)

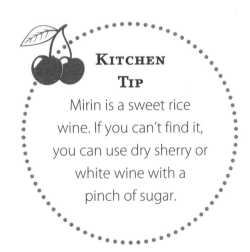

KITCHEN TIP

Mirin is a sweet rice wine. If you can't find it, you can use dry sherry or white wine with a pinch of sugar.

1. Preheat the oven to 350°F.
2. Place the carrot, parsnip, and squash in a large bowl with the rosemary. Add 3 tablespoons of the oil and toss to coat. Sprinkle with salt and pepper. Arrange on a baking sheet in a single layer and roast for 20 to 25 minutes, until soft but not mushy.
3. In a small saucepan over medium heat, combine the stock and wine and heat to simmering. Lower the temperature to a simmer.
4. In a large nonstick pot, heat the remaining 2 tablespoons of olive oil over medium heat. Add the garlic, onion, and rice and sauté for 3 to 5 minutes, or until the rice starts to be toasted.
5. Add 1 cup of the simmering broth-and-wine mixture to the rice and cook, stirring continuously, until the liquid is mostly absorbed. Continue adding the broth 1 cup at a time, cooking and stirring as it is absorbed. It will take about 20 minutes for all the broth to be absorbed and for the rice to become tender and creamy.
6. Add the almond milk, tahini, nutritional yeast, lemon juice, and mirin and cook for a further 5 minutes. Stir in the roasted veggies. Season to taste with salt and pepper.

Sushi in a Bowl

SERVES 4

Mayim makes avocado sushi for her sons at home, because it is one of their favorite foods and it gets expensive to keep ordering it in restaurants by the dozen. One night at home, we put all the ingredients in a bowl and voilà: Sushi in a Bowl was born. The rice vinegar is optional, but it gives a sweet and sushilike consistency and taste. You can use any rice, but for the most authentic sticky consistency, use Japanese white rice labeled "sushi rice."

1 cup white sushi rice
1 tablespoon rice vinegar
1 avocado, peeled, pitted, and diced
1 tablespoon sesame seeds or gomasio (see Kitchen Tip)
¼ cup shredded nori (optional)

1. Prepare the sushi rice according to the package directions. Place in a large bowl. Drizzle with the rice vinegar and add the avocado. Sprinkle the sesame seeds on top, or sprinkle with shredded nori, if desired.

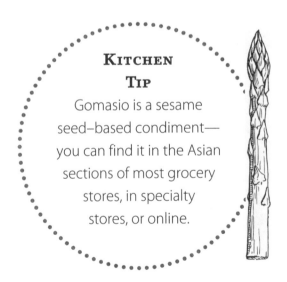

KITCHEN TIP

Gomasio is a sesame seed–based condiment— you can find it in the Asian sections of most grocery stores, in specialty stores, or online.

Udon with Edamame and Peanut Sauce

SERVES 4

A wonderful alternative to plain pasta and marinara sauce, here is a sweet but nutritious noodle dish with peanut sauce and edamame. The sauce can be made ahead of time and kept in a sealed bottle in the refrigerator. Carrots, bell peppers, and celery add extra crunch and color.

PEANUT SAUCE
½ cup smooth peanut butter
¼ cup low-sodium soy sauce
⅓ cup warm water
2 tablespoons fresh ginger, peeled and chopped
2 garlic cloves, peeled
2 tablespoons unseasoned rice vinegar
1½ tablespoons sesame oil
1 tablespoon agave nectar
¼ bunch fresh cilantro

1 (8-ounce) package udon noodles, cooked according to the package directions
1 cup cooked edamame
1 cup carrot, grated
1 cup cucumber, diced
1 cup bean sprouts
1 red bell pepper, seeded and diced (about ½ cup)
¼ cup roasted peanuts, chopped, for garnish
⅛ cup fresh cilantro, chopped, for garnish

1. Place all the ingredients for the sauce in a blender or a food processor, and puree.
2. In a large bowl, toss the noodles with the sauce, then top with the veggies.
3. Garnish with the peanuts and cilantro.

Thai Pasta

SERVES 4

Mayim's Aunt Linda introduced her to this recipe, and her boys ask for it again and again. The marinade is the secret: a combination of sesame oil, soy sauce, and agave nectar makes the dish sweet and subtle. The red pepper flakes provide an optional hint of spice, and we added some vegetables to up the nutrition quotient. If you double this recipe or more, do not let the corn oil exceed ½ cup or it will be too oily.

12 ounces linguine or spaghetti, cooked according to the package directions

2 teaspoons vegetable oil

1 teaspoon toasted sesame oil

1 (6-ounce) package button mushrooms or baby bellas

1 red bell pepper, seeded and diced

2 baby bok choy, chopped, or 2 cups spinach, chopped

1 cup carrot, shredded (about 3 large carrots)

SAUCE

¼ cup corn oil

3 tablespoons sesame oil

3 tablespoons agave nectar or maple syrup

2 tablespoons soy sauce

1 tablespoon red pepper flakes (optional)

¼ cup fresh cilantro, chopped, for garnish

3 scallions, sliced, for garnish

½ cup peanuts, chopped, for garnish

1. Place the cooked pasta in a large serving bowl.
2. Heat the vegetable and sesame oils in a large skillet over high heat. Add the mushrooms, bell pepper, bok choy, and carrot and sauté until the bok choy is wilted, 2 to 3 minutes. Add to the cooked pasta.
3. To make the sauce, mix together the corn oil, sesame oil, agave nectar or maple syrup, soy sauce, and red pepper flakes in a small bowl. Pour into the pasta and veggies and toss to coat. Add the cilantro, scallions, and peanuts and mix.

Daiya-Style Pizza

MAKES 2 PIZZAS; SERVES 4

Everyone loves pizza, and this homemade crust will make you wonder why you don't have pizza more often. The crust could not be easier to make, and when topped with Daiya nondairy cheese (the best cheese we have found for melty gooey awesome pizza), you will feel like you are at your favorite pizzeria.

CRUST

1 (0.25-ounce) package regular or quick-acting active dry yeast

1 cup warm water

2½ cups all-purpose flour

2 tablespoons olive oil, plus more for oiling pan

½ teaspoon salt

Cornmeal, for sprinkling

TOPPINGS (SEE ALSO VARIATIONS)

Your vegan sauce of choice

1 (8-ounce) package Daiya cheese

¼ cup olives (optional)

½ cup onion, sliced, or bell pepper, seeded (optional)

2 teaspoons garlic, minced (optional)

1. Dissolve the yeast in the warm water in a medium bowl. Stir in the flour, 2 tablespoons of the olive oil, and the salt. Beat vigorously, about 20 strokes. Cover and let rest for 20 minutes.
2. Preheat the oven to 425°F. Grease two cookie sheets or 12-inch pizza pans with olive oil and sprinkle with the cornmeal.
3. Remove the dough from the bowl. Place half of the dough on a clean, floured countertop. With floured fingers, pat into an 11-inch circle. Repeat with the other half of the dough and transfer each circle to one of the prepared pans. Prick each dough circle all over with a fork. Bake for 10 minutes on lower rack, or until just starting to brown.

4. Remove the pans from the oven. Add your desired sauce and toppings and bake for 10 to 15 more minutes, until the cheese melts.

VARIATIONS: Creative toppings for pizzas:

- Mushrooms, sun-dried tomato, and olives
- Mushrooms, pineapple, and caramelized onion
- Arugula, figs, and CASHEW CHEESE (SEE NEXT PAGE)
- Vegan sausage, peppers, and onion

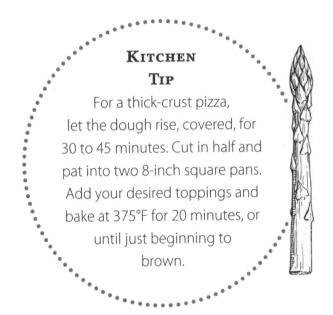

KITCHEN TIP

For a thick-crust pizza, let the dough rise, covered, for 30 to 45 minutes. Cut in half and pat into two 8-inch square pans. Add your desired toppings and bake at 375°F for 20 minutes, or until just beginning to brown.

Cashew Cheese

MAKES 1 CUP CHEESE

Here's a cashew-based cheese to use on pizza.

1 cup raw cashews
Juice of ½ lemon
1 tablespoon nutritional yeast
Salt and freshly ground black pepper

1. Soak the cashews in 1 cup of water for at least 2 hours. Drain. Place the cashews, lemon juice, and nutritional yeast in a blender and blend until smooth, adding 1 tablespoon of water at a time, or up to 1 cup, to make the cashew mixture creamy but not runny. Season to taste with salt and pepper. Refrigerate until cool.

VARIATION: To make herbed cashew cheese, add 2 tablespoons of chopped fresh rosemary and 2 tablespoons of chopped fresh dill, stirring them in with a spoon.

Veggie Chili

SERVES 8

This is a delicious one-pot speedy meal inspired by Mayim's friend Denise, the photographer for this book. It's a smart recipe to double, since it keeps well in the freezer for months and can be defrosted any time for a super healthy, satisfying, and easy meal. We serve it with a variety of toppings, such as vegan sour cream, diced onion, and avocado. We also like to pair it with homemade CREAMED CORN BREAD (PAGE 166).

This is great to serve at parties, and Denise and Mayim take it in its frozen form on camping trips. They let it defrost the first night and heat it up for a communal hearty meal on the second night.

¼ cup vegetable oil

½ head garlic, peeled and minced

1 large onion, chopped

3 celery stalks, chopped

3 carrots, chopped

1 bell pepper, seeded and chopped

1 medium-size zucchini, chopped

2 cups kale, chopped (optional)

½ cup fresh cilantro, chopped

2 tablespoons chili powder

1 tablespoon ground cumin

1 tablespoon garlic powder

1 tablespoon freshly ground black pepper

2 teaspoons salt

2 (14-ounce) cans tomato sauce

2 (6-ounce) cans tomato paste

1 tablespoon maple syrup

2 (14-ounce) cans kidney beans, drained and rinsed

2 (14-ounce) cans black beans, drained and rinsed

2 (14-ounce) cans pinto beans, drained and rinsed

½ (12-ounce) bag frozen corn kernels

1. In a large pot, heat the oil over medium-high heat and sauté the garlic, onion, celery, carrots, pepper, zucchini, and kale, if using, (but *not* the corn) just until softened, about 10 minutes.

2. Add all the herbs, spices, and salt and cook for 5 more minutes. Add the tomato sauce, tomato paste, and maple syrup and stir for 3 more minutes. Add the beans and stir for 3 minutes. Add the corn and simmer for 15 to 20 minutes.

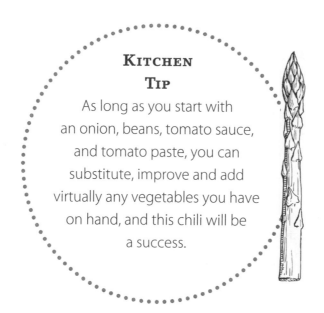

KITCHEN TIP

As long as you start with an onion, beans, tomato sauce, and tomato paste, you can substitute, improve and add virtually any vegetables you have on hand, and this chili will be a success.

Creamy Enchilada Casserole

SERVES 4

Mexican dishes, such as enchiladas, can be hard to veganize because of the amount of cheese typically called for. This recipe solves that problem with a simple vegan cheese sauce and a delicious simple filling. We like to use sprouted or whole wheat tortillas to line this casserole, and we serve it with vegan sour cream, extra salsa, and diced avocado.

This is a great meal for large groups, and it freezes well for easy reheating.

Nonstick cooking spray

BEAN FILLING
1 tablespoon olive oil
1 small onion, chopped
1 garlic clove, minced
1 (14-ounce) can pinto, kidney, or black beans, drained and rinsed
1 (16-ounce) can vegan refried beans
½ cup mild or medium-hot salsa
2 tablespoons fresh cilantro, finely chopped
½ teaspoon drled oregano

CHEESE SAUCE
1 ¼ cups plain unsweetened almond, rice, or soy milk
2 tablespoons unbleached all-purpose flour
1 cup grated vegan cheese, Daiya preferred

8 to 10 (6-inch) sprouted or whole wheat tortillas, cut into quarters
1 scallion, thinly sliced

1. Preheat the oven to 400°F. Lightly oil a shallow round 2-quart casserole or a 9 × 13-inch baking pan with the nonstick cooking spray.

2. To make the bean filling, heat the oil in a medium skillet over medium heat. Add the onion and sauté until translucent, about 5 minutes. Add the garlic and continue to sauté until the onion is golden. Stir in the remaining filling ingredients and cook until the filling is heated through, about 5 minutes.

3. To make the cheese sauce, heat 1 cup of the nondairy milk in a small saucepan. In a small bowl, whisk the flour into the remaining milk and then whisk it into the saucepan. Sprinkle in the vegan cheese. Bring the sauce to a gentle simmer, stirring frequently, and cook until thickened, about 7 minutes.

4. Line the prepared pan with a single layer of tortillas. Pour in the filling and spread evenly over the tortillas. Cover with the remaining tortilla pieces. Pour the cheese sauce evenly over the tortillas, then add scallions on top.

5. Bake for 15 minutes, or until the cheese is bubbly.

Build-Your-Own
Black Bean and Quinoa Tacos

SERVES 4

Build-it-yourself meals are a great way to feed vegan kids, because they can put in everything they like and leave out what they don't. Giving kids options is often a way to take the pressure off at mealtimes if there have been struggles about food. More often than not, kids love eating meals they help put together.

BLACK BEANS
Nonstick cooking spray

1 cup onion, chopped

2 medium-size green or red bell peppers, seeded and diced (about 1½ cups)

2 medium-size zucchini, chopped (about 1½ cups)

2 teaspoons garlic, minced

2 tablespoons olive oil

1 teaspoon Cajun or Old Bay seasoning

1 teaspoon ground cumin

1 (14-ounce) can black beans, drained and rinsed

1 cup frozen corn

QUINOA
1 cup cooked quinoa

2 medium-size tomatoes, diced

¼ cup fresh cilantro, chopped

½ cup scallions, finely sliced

Juice of 2 limes

1 teaspoon salt

½ teaspoon freshly ground black pepper

1 cup shredded vegan cheese, Daiya preferred (optional)

8 tortillas

TACO ADD-INS

1 cup shredded cheese, Daiya preferred

½ cup tomatoes, diced

1 cup GUACAMOLE (PAGE 110) or 1 cup avocado, peeled and sliced

1 cup frozen corn, thawed and drained

½ cup vegan sour cream

1 (8-ounce) container fresh vegan salsa

1. Preheat the oven to 350°F. Spray a 9-inch baking dish with cooking spray.

2. To make the black beans, in a 10-inch skillet over medium heat, sauté the onion, peppers, zucchini, and garlic in oil until soft, about 7 minutes. Add the Cajun or Old Bay seasoning and cumin and sauté for another 2 minutes. Add the beans and corn and cook for another 2 minutes. Pour into the prepared baking dish.

3. To make the quinoa, in a large bowl, mix together the cooked quinoa, tomatoes, cilantro, scallions, lime juice, salt, and pepper. Spread the quinoa and tomatoes on top of the beans. Sprinkle with vegan cheese, if using.

4. Bake for 10 to 15 minutes, or until the cheese is melted.

5. Serve along with bowls of taco add-ins, and let people add what they wish on heated tortillas.

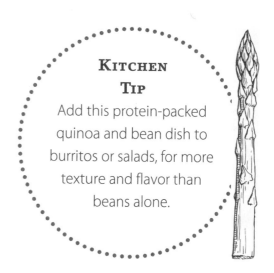

KITCHEN TIP

Add this protein-packed quinoa and bean dish to burritos or salads, for more texture and flavor than beans alone.

Vegetable and Tofu Curry

SERVES 4

Curry can be overpowering, especially for young kids or those with a delicate palate. This recipe is subtle without being bland, and it allows for substitutions, depending on what vegetables you like. Serve over rice or udon noodles.

2 tablespoons canola oil

1 large yellow onion, finely chopped

4 medium-size garlic cloves, minced

1 (2-inch) piece fresh ginger, peeled and finely grated (about 1 tablespoon)

1 tablespoon ground coriander

1½ teaspoons ground cumin

¾ teaspoon turmeric

½ teaspoon cayenne pepper

1 tablespoon tomato paste

2 cups vegan vegetable stock

1 (3-inch) cinnamon stick

1 teaspoon fine sea salt

¼ teaspoon freshly ground black pepper

1 small cauliflower, cut into 1½-inch florets (about 2 cups)

1 pound sweet potatoes, peeled and cut into 1-inch cubes (2 to 3 cups)

1 (14-ounce) package extra-firm sprouted tofu, cut into ¼-inch cubes

4 medium-size tomatoes, cored, seeded, and coarsely chopped (about 1½ cups)

2 large carrots, peeled and diced (about 1½ cups)

2 tablespoons freshly squeezed lime juice

2 tablespoons fresh cilantro, chopped, for garnish

1. In a large pot, heat the oil over medium-high heat. Add the onion and cook, stirring occasionally, until beginning to brown, 3 to 4 minutes. Lower the heat to medium and cook until the onion is browned, about 5 more minutes. Add the garlic and ginger and cook, stirring, for 1 minute, to blend the flavors. Add the coriander, cumin, turmeric, and cayenne and cook for another minute.

Add the tomato paste and stir until blended. Add the stock, cinnamon stick, salt, and pepper and bring to a boil. Lower the heat to medium-low and simmer for 10 minutes.

2. Add the cauliflower, sweet potatoes, sprouted tofu, tomatoes, and carrots. Raise the heat to medium-high and return to a boil. Lower the heat to simmer, cover, and cook for 20 to 25 minutes, until the vegetables are soft. Discard the cinnamon stick. Stir in the lime juice. Season to taste with salt. Serve garnished with the cilantro.

Spanikopita with Yogurt Dipping Sauce

MAKES 24 SPANIKOPITA; SERVES 8 AS AN APPETIZER

Greek and Mediterranean dishes often feature delicious fillings hidden in phyllo dough. This vegan version of cheese and spinach pockets tastes like the real deal. They make a wonderful party food. The folding takes a few tries (the triangles are folded as you would fold a flag), but once you get the hang of it, you will be making these more and more. Serve with a vegan yogurt sauce for authentic dipping.

1 (12-ounce) box frozen spinach, thawed and drained well
1 ¼ cups RAW NUT CHEESE, ricotta-style (see PAGE 111)
1 (16-ounce) package whole wheat phyllo dough, thawed
Vegetable oil, to seal

YOGURT DIPPING SAUCE
1 cup unsweetened soy yogurt
½ cup vegan sour cream
2 cucumbers, peeled, seeded, sliced into rounds, then each round cut into 4 wedges
3 garlic cloves, minced
2 tablespoons olive oil
2 tablespoons freshly squeezed lemon juice
1 teaspoon salt
2 tablespoons fresh dill, chopped, or 1 tablespoon dried

1. Preheat the oven to 350°F. Combine the spinach with the raw nut cheese in a medium bowl.
2. Keep the dough moist as you work by covering with a moist cloth, and cut the phyllo into four strips per sheet of phyllo.
3. Place a generous tablespoon of filling at the top of a strip of phyllo and fold over into a triangle. Continue folding into triangles until you seal the edge by brushing it with oil. Repeat to make twenty-four triangles.
4. Place each triangle on a large baking sheet and bake for 20 to 25 minutes, until the edges start to brown.
5. To make the sauce, mix all the ingredients together in a medium bowl and refrigerate for 30 minutes to let the flavors meld.

Zucchini Pie

SERVES 6

Mayim's Uncle Loren grew amazing zucchini in his San Francisco backyard. Over the years, he found tons of great recipes to use them in. This recipe combines zucchini with onion and grated vegan cheese and not much else, but the flavor is dynamite. The whole wheat crust doesn't even need to be rolled out; just combine the ingredients and press into a pie pan. If you want, call it "Zucchini Pizza" instead of "Zucchini Pie"; you'll be amazed at how many more people try it with the word pizza *in the title!*

CRUST
1 cup whole wheat flour
½ teaspoon salt
6 tablespoons vegan margarine
2 tablespoons cold water

1 tablespoon olive oil
1 onion, chopped
4 medium-size zucchini, coarsely grated
Egg replacer equivalent of 2 eggs
1 cup nondairy cheese, mozzarella style, Daiya preferred, grated
1 tablespoon Dijon mustard (optional)

1. Preheat the oven to 350°F. Place the flour and salt in a large bowl. Add the margarine, cutting it in until the dough is crumbly. Add the cold water. Mix lightly and form into a ball.
2. Press the ball of dough into an 8-inch pie pan until it covers the bottom and up the sides to the top of the pan.
3. Heat the oil in a large skillet over medium-high heat. Sauté the onion for about 5 minutes, or until soft.
4. Spread the mustard on the bottom of the pie shell. Mix the zucchini, onion, vegan cheese, and egg replacer together in a large bowl and pour over the crust.
5. Bake for 45 minutes to 1 hour, until the crust starts to brown and the cheese starts to set.

Shepherd's Pie

SERVES 4

Mayim and her sons had never tasted shepherd's pie until they had this one, which was crafted by Mayim's friend and contributing chef, Ali. They ate the entire batch in one sitting! Who needs a meat version, when the combination of lentils, vegetables, and spices makes for such an incredible blend of vegan tastes? (You can also substitute chickpeas for half of the lentils.)

Nonstick cooking spray

4 large russet potatoes, peeled and diced

½ cup plain, unsweetened nondairy milk

¼ cup vegan margarine

2 teaspoons salt

¾ teaspoon freshly ground black pepper

2 tablespoons olive oil

½ cup onion, chopped

½ cup celery, chopped

½ cup carrot, chopped

1 teaspoon garlic, minced

2 teaspoons dried Italian herb seasoning

2 (14-ounce) cans lentils, drained and rinsed

1 cup frozen peas

1 tablespoon vegan Worcestershire sauce

2 teaspoons Dijon mustard

1. Preheat the oven to 350°F. Oil a 9-inch baking pan with the cooking spray.
2. Boil the potatoes in salted water until tender, about 20 minutes. Drain, return them to the pot, and mash.
3. Place the nondairy milk and margarine in a small saucepan over medium heat and cook until the margarine has melted. Add 1 teaspoon of the salt and ½ teaspoon of the pepper, and then add to the mashed potatoes and stir well until incorporated.

4. In a large pan over high heat, heat the oil and sauté the onion, celery, carrot, and garlic until soft, about 8 minutes. Add the Italian seasoning and cook for 30 seconds. Add the lentils, peas, Worcestershire sauce, mustard, and the remaining teaspoon of salt and ¼ teaspoon of pepper and cook for a further 5 minutes.

5. Pour into the prepared pan and spread the mashed potato on top. Bake for 30 minutes, until golden.

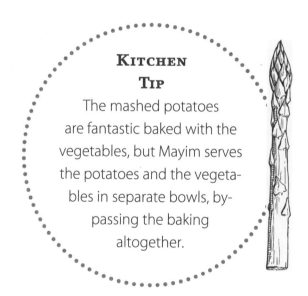

KITCHEN TIP

The mashed potatoes are fantastic baked with the vegetables, but Mayim serves the potatoes and the vegetables in separate bowls, bypassing the baking altogether.

CHAPTER 10

Breads

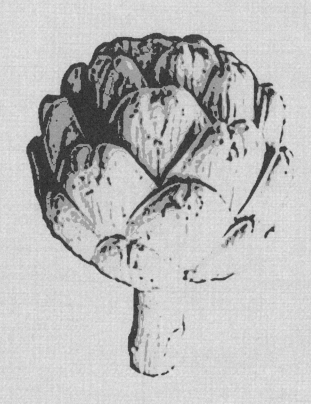

Creamed Corn Bread

SERVES 8

Corn bread is tempting to eat on its own, but we like it with such dishes as chili. This creamy and sweet corn bread recipe is Mayim's and contributing friend Chef Ali's; she hails from South Africa, but you wouldn't know she wasn't from the American South from the authentic taste of this amazing corn bread.

$^2/_3$ cup maple syrup
$^1/_3$ cup canola oil
1 cup plain, unsweetened soy milk
1 cup whole wheat flour
1 cup cornmeal
1 tablespoon baking powder
1 teaspoon salt
1 cup creamed corn
1 cup frozen corn kernels

1. Preheat the oven to 350°F. In a medium bowl, mix together the maple syrup, oil, and soy milk.
2. In a large bowl, whisk together the flour, cornmeal, baking powder, and salt.
3. Pour the wet ingredients into the dry and mix together. Stir in the creamed corn and corn kernels and pour into a greased 9-inch square pan. Bake for about 35 minutes, or until a toothpick inserted into the center comes out clean.

Pumpkin Bread

SERVES 6 TO 8

When October rolls around, many of us crave creative pumpkin-inspired recipes. This one calls for pumpkin pie filling, and makes a dark, sweet, and gently spiced bread. Serve it with autumn meals or as a breakfast treat.

½ cup canola oil, plus more for pan

1 cup vegan pumpkin pie mix

¾ cup granulated sugar

½ cup light molasses

1 teaspoon vanilla extract

2 cups all-purpose flour

1½ teaspoons baking powder

½ teaspoon baking soda

¾ teaspoon kosher salt

1 teaspoon ground cinnamon

¼ teaspoon ground nutmeg

¼ teaspoon ground cloves

½ teaspoon ground ginger

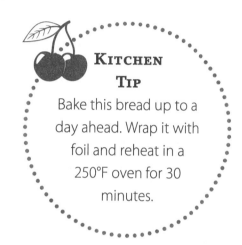

KITCHEN TIP

Bake this bread up to a day ahead. Wrap it with foil and reheat in a 250°F oven for 30 minutes.

1. Preheat the oven to 350°F. Oil a 9 × 5-inch loaf pan.
2. In a large bowl, combine the oil, pumpkin pie mix, sugar, molasses, and vanilla. In a medium bowl, combine the flour, baking powder, baking soda, salt, cinnamon, nutmeg, cloves, and ginger. Slowly stir the dry ingredients into the pumpkin mixture. Pour into the prepared pan.
3. Bake for 60 to 65 minutes, until a toothpick inserted into the center comes out clean. Transfer the pan to a wire rack for 10 minutes.
4. Using a knife, loosen the bread from the pan. Invert it onto a cutting board. Serve warm.

Turtle Bread

MAKES 1 LOAF; SERVES 4

We have yet to find an easier and faster-to-make bread than this one. The fact that it can be shaped to look like a turtle makes it even better. Kids can help mix it, shape it, and decorate it, and the taste is fantastic, especially considering how little work it requires.

2½ to 3 cups all-purpose flour
1 (0.25-ounce) envelope quick-acting active dry yeast
1 tablespoon sugar
1 teaspoon salt
⅓ cup almond milk (soy or rice milk works fine, too)
1 tablespoon vegan margarine
Egg replacer equivalent of 1 egg
2 raisins
Vegetable or canola oil, for pan

1. Preheat the oven to 400°F. Mix 1½ cups of the flour, and the yeast, sugar, and salt in a large bowl.
2. Place the nondairy milk and margarine in a small saucepan over medium heat. Add ½ cup of water and heat until the margarine has melted, 125° to 130°F. Stir into the dry ingredients. Stir in the egg replacer. Add enough flour by the half-cup to make the dough easy to handle.
3. Transfer the dough to a floured surface and knead until smooth and elastic, about 5 minutes. Cover with a clean dish towel and let rest for 10 minutes.

KITCHEN TIP

For braided challah-style bread, follow the instructions but braid the dough, using 3 ropes of the same length and thickness. Bake as indicated until golden brown.

4. Lightly grease a cookie sheet. Pull off a piece of dough and roll into a 2-inch ball for the head. Shape 5 additional walnut-size pieces of dough into balls for feet and a tail. Shape the remaining dough into a ball for the body. Place the body on the prepared cookie sheet and flatten slightly. Attach the head, feet, and tail by placing an end of each under the edge of the body to secure it. Press the raisins into head for eyes. Cover with a cloth and let rise for 20 minutes.

5. Make crisscross cuts in the body, ¼-inch deep, to look like a turtle shell. Bake until golden brown, 20 to 25 minutes.

NOTE: *This bread freezes well, so make extra batches for defrosting later.*

Olive Walnut Bread

This bread takes a little effort, but the results are so professional we think it's worth it. Olive-walnut bread is perfect with vegan cheese spreads, tapenades, or simply accompanying a festive meal.

Bake this bread on a ceramic baking stone, if you have one.

½ cup nondairy milk, such as soy or rice milk

1½ teaspoons active dry yeast

About 10 ounces green olives

¼ cup olive oil, plus more for greasing bowl

½ teaspoon salt

1 cup whole wheat pastry flour

About 3 cups unbleached all-purpose flour

Egg replacer equivalent of 1 egg

1. Place the nondairy milk and ½ cup of water in a small saucepan over medium heat, and heat to body temperature. Remove from the heat and transfer to a large bowl. Stir in the yeast, and leave for 10 minutes, or until foamy.

2. Set aside 8 of the olives. Remove the pits by pressing down hard with the heel of your palm. For stubborn ones, use a paring knife to cut out the pit. Chop the pitted olives coarsely. You should have about 1 cup.

3. Stir in the chopped olives, ¼ cup of the olive oil, and the salt and whole wheat flour to make a smooth batter, then add the all-purpose flour until the dough is too stiff to handle.

4. Turn out the dough onto a floured surface and knead for 5 minutes, adding more flour when it sticks. You won't be able to get the dough silky smooth because of the olives, but work it until it has a nice even consistency.

5. Grease a bowl with olive oil and add the dough. Rub a little oil on the top of the dough, Cover the bowl with plastic wrap and set it aside to rise for an hour or so, in a warm place.

6. Once it has doubled in bulk, punch it down, and then turn it out onto the counter. Divide the dough into 3 pieces. Roll each piece into a rope about 22

inches long and ¾-inch wide. Make a tight braid, then form the braid into a spiral, with the edges of the dough just touching. (The dough will rise upward, not just outward.) Set the dough aside to rise on a baking stone, or place the dough directly on a cookie sheet. Cover the bread lightly with a clean dish towel and set aside to rise, about 1 hour.

7. Preheat the oven to 400°F. Insert the baking stone, if you're using one.

8. Brush the bread with some of the beaten egg replacer and firmly lodge the remaining olives in the bread, in any pattern you like. Slide the bread onto the hot baking stone or place the cookie sheet into the oven. Continue baking until the bread is nicely colored all over, about 45 minutes. Set the bread on a wire rack to cool.

Bev's Banana Bread

SERVES 8

Mayim's mother has been making this banana bread for as long as Mayim can remember. This updated version substitutes agave nectar for the sugar and egg replacer for the eggs without losing any of the flavor. We like almonds instead of walnuts for a crunchier bread, and you can also add ½ cup of vegan chocolate chips for a sweet option, or ½ cup of blueberries for a colorful version. This recipe uses no fat at all!

Nonstick cooking spray

3 ripe bananas

Egg replacer equivalent of 2 eggs

2 cups all-purpose flour

¾ cup agave nectar

1 teaspoon salt

1 teaspoon baking soda

½ cup walnuts, chopped

KITCHEN TIP

For a heartier bread, add ¼ to ½ cup of wheat germ, ground flaxseeds, or rolled oats, reducing the flour by the same amount. Also makes great muffins, prepared as directed and poured into an oiled muffin pan.

1. Preheat the oven to 350°F. Oil a 9 × 5-inch loaf pan with the nonstick cooking spray.
2. Mash the bananas in a large bowl. Add the egg replacer and stir to combine. Add the remaining ingredients, mix well, and pour into the prepared pan. Bake for 1 hour, until a toothpick inserted into the center comes out clean.

Soft Pretzels

MAKES 8 MEDIUM-SIZE PRETZELS

Soft pretzels bring the fun of pretzels at the circus, the movies, or the county fair to your home, in a vegan version. Sprinkle them with kosher salt, cinnamon and sugar, or anything else you like.

1 (0.25-ounce) envelope active dry yeast
1½ cups lukewarm water (100°F)
¾ teaspoon salt
1½ teaspoons sugar
4 cups all-purpose flour
¼ cup soy milk

1. Preheat the oven to 425°F. In a large bowl, dissolve the yeast in the lukewarm water. Mix in the salt and sugar, and then mix in the flour.
2. Turn out the dough onto a floured surface and knead until soft and smooth.
3. Cut the dough into 4 equal pieces. Roll each piece into a rope about 4 inches long and shape into circles, because making a pretzel shape hurts our brains! If you want the classic pretzel shape, look at a picture of a pretzel and try to imitate it!
4. Place the pretzels about an inch or two apart on a parchment-lined baking sheet. Brush with the soy milk and bake for 25 minutes.

Hot Pretzel Challah Bread

MAKES 2 LOAVES CHALLAH; SERVES 8

Challah is the traditional braided Jewish bread served on the Sabbath and Holy Days. It is known for its crusty exterior and soft and slightly sweet inside.

A vegan company in Los Angeles makes a pretzel challah that is not only crusty on the outside, but tastes like the best soft pretzel ever. This recipe takes a little bit of work to get the crust just right, but it will not disappoint! It's best eaten warm on the day it's made, as the outer crust can get hard the next day. Dip in pretzel salt or kosher salt and add sesame seeds, if you like. Serve with mustard.

1 tablespoon active dry yeast

6 teaspoons sugar

¼ cup lukewarm water

¾ teaspoon kosher salt

⅛ cup canola oil, plus more for bowl

3 cups bread flour

⅔ cup baking soda

Salt or sesame seeds, for sprinkling

1. Preheat the oven to 350°F. In a medium glass bowl or measuring cup, combine the yeast, 1½ teaspoons of the sugar, and the lukewarm water. Leave for 10 minutes, or until foamy.
2. Meanwhile, in the bowl of a stand mixer fitted with a dough hook, on medium-low speed, mix the remaining 4½ teaspoons of sugar, 1 cup of water, and the kosher salt and oil. (This also can be done by hand with a whisk.)
3. Add the yeast mixture to the mixing bowl, beating well. With the mixer on low speed, add the flour. Raise the speed to medium and knead for 4 to 5 minutes, until a smooth, satiny dough forms. It will have almost a matte finish. If you are kneading in the flour by hand, it may take a few minutes longer to get a good, smooth texture. Place in a lightly oiled bowl, cover with a clean dish towel and allow the dough to rise in a warm place for 1½ hours, or until doubled in size.
4. Line a baking sheet with parchment paper.

5. Transfer the dough to a lightly floured surface. If the dough is sticky, knead in more flour, a little bit at a time, until the dough is easy to roll. Divide the dough into six equal balls and roll each into a long strand. Braid three strands of dough into a challah, for a total of two challahs. Place on the prepared baking sheet.

6. Bring 8 cups of water and the baking soda to a boil in a pot with a wide opening. Gently and carefully, lower a challah into the baking soda solution. Using two wooden spoons or spatulas, carefully turn the challah so both sides get equally covered in the water, or bathe the top with spoonfuls of the solution. Remove after 30 seconds and place back on the parchment-lined pan. Repeat with the other challah.

7. Brush the top of each challah with some water from the pot and then top with salt or sesame seeds.

8. Bake for 30 minutes, or until starting to brown.

CHAPTER 11

Desserts

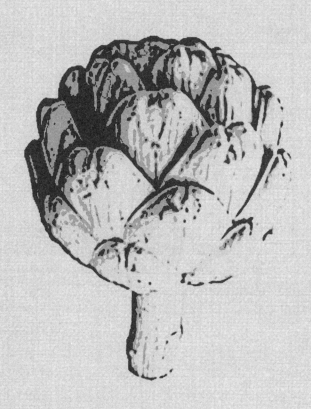

Chocolate Chip Pumpkin Cookies

This recipe makes fluffy cookies with the spice and warmth of pumpkin and the sweetness and delectable temptation of chocolate. They are especially fun around the time when pumpkins are arranged on doorsteps.

Nonstick cooking spray

8 tablespoons (1 stick) unsalted vegan margarine, at room temperature

¾ cup brown sugar

¾ cup granulated sugar

1 cup canned pure pumpkin

Egg replacer equivalent of 1 egg

2 teaspoons vanilla extract

2½ cups all-purpose flour

1 teaspoon ground cinnamon

½ teaspoon ground ginger

¼ teaspoon ground cloves

Pinch of ground nutmeg

Pinch of mace (optional)

1 teaspoon baking powder

1 teaspoon baking soda

½ teaspoon salt

1 cup vegan semisweet chocolate chips

1. Preheat the oven to 350°F. Spray two baking sheets with the cooking spray.
2. In a large bowl, mix the margarine and sugars until creamy. Add the pumpkin and mix well. Then add the egg replacer and mix well. Finally, add the vanilla and stir to combine.
3. Stir together the dry ingredients in a separate bowl. Add the dry ingredients to the pumpkin mixture, and stir to combine. Fold in the chocolate chips with a spoon or spatula.
4. Spoon the batter in ¼-cup measures onto the prepared baking sheets, leaving 1 inch between cookies. Bake for 15 minutes, or until lightly golden brown. Let the cookies rest on the pan for 1 minute after removing them from the oven, and then let cool on a wire rack.

Deep Dark Chocolate Cookies

Specialty vegan cookies can be a challenge to master, so when we perfected this vegan version of the classic "cracked top" chocolate cookie, we were thrilled. They take a little work, but the richness and beauty of these cookies make it so worth it.

Nonstick cooking spray

1½ cups vegan bittersweet chocolate chips

Egg replacer equivalent of 1 egg

2½ cups confectioners' sugar

½ cup natural unsweetened cocoa powder

1 tablespoon cornstarch

¼ teaspoon salt

1. Preheat the oven to 400°F. Spray two large baking sheets with the cooking spray.
2. Melt 1 cup of the chocolate chips in a small glass bowl in the microwave, stirring twice, about 2 minutes. Stir until the chocolate is completely melted. Let cool for about 5 minutes.
3. Place the egg replacer in a small bowl, and gradually beat 1 cup of the confectioners' sugar into it. Continue beating until the mixture resembles soft marshmallow creme, 2 to 3 minutes.
4. In a medium bowl, whisk together 1 cup of the sugar and the cocoa, cornstarch, and salt.
5. With an electric mixer on low speed, beat the dry ingredients into the egg replacer mixture.
6. Stir in the lukewarm chocolate and remaining ½ cup of chocolate chips (the dough will become very stiff).
7. Place the remaining ½ cup of confectioners' sugar in a shallow bowl. Roll rounded tablespoonfuls of the dough into balls. Roll the balls in the sugar, coating thickly. Place the cookie balls 2 inches apart on the prepared baking sheets. Bake until puffed and the tops crack, about 10 minutes.
8. Leaving the cookies on the baking sheets, let the pans cool on a wire rack for about 10 minutes. Transfer the cookies to racks and let cool completely, about 30 minutes.

"Cream Cheese" Walnut Cookies

Mayim wanted to veganize this recipe for years, and she finally figured it out, with tremendous results. These cookies may not win a prize for healthiest cookie on the block, but they may win for the tastiest.

1 pound (4 sticks) vegan margarine, at room temperature

6 ounces vegan cream cheese, at room temperature

1¼ cups sugar

2 tablespoons plus ½ teaspoon vanilla extract

4 cups all-purpose flour

1½ teaspoons salt

2½ cups walnuts, chopped and toasted

1. Preheat the oven to 350°F. Line two baking sheets with parchment paper.
2. In a small bowl, whisk together the flour and salt.
3. Using a rimmed baking sheet, toast the walnuts for 8 to 10 minutes, watching closely. You could also use a toaster oven until the walnuts start to darken, or sauté without oil in a small pan until they brown and become fragrant, about 5 minutes. Remove and set aside.
4. Blend the margarine and cream cheese until pale and fluffy. Add the sugar and vanilla. Mix for another 2 to 3 minutes. Add the flour and salt, and then add 1½ cups of the toasted walnuts.
5. Transfer the dough to a clean floured surface and divide it in half. Shape each piece into a log about 8 inches long and 2 inches wide. Wrap each piece in parchment paper and freeze for 30 minutes.
6. Remove the dough from the freezer. Unwrap each log and roll in the remaining 1 cup of walnuts. Cut the logs into ¼-inch rounds and place about 1 inch apart on the prepared baking sheets.
7. Bake for 18 to 20 minutes, until the cookies are golden around the edges, rotating the cookies halfway through. To rotate the cookies effectively, turn the pans and switch the trays to the other oven racks. Remove from the oven and let cool on a wire rack.

Oatmeal Cookies

MAKES 24 COOKIES

The comfort of an oatmeal cookie is timeless. This vegan version calls for lots of margarine, but the result is a smooth and delightful cookie. Use raisins for a traditional version or vegan chocolate chips for a sweeter one.

16 tablespoons (2 sticks) vegan margarine, at room temperature
1¼ cups brown sugar
Egg replacer equivalent of 2 eggs
2 cups rolled oats
2 cups all-purpose flour
1½ teaspoons vanilla extract
1 teaspoon salt
1 teaspoon ground cinnamon
1 teaspoon baking soda
½ cup raisins or vegan chocolate chips

1. Preheat the oven to 350°F. In a large bowl, mix the margarine with the sugar until creamy. Mix in the egg replacer and ⅓ cup of water. Add the remaining ingredients and stir to combine.
2. Drop by heaping tablespoonfuls 1 inch apart onto an ungreased baking sheet and bake for 15 minutes, until starting to brown. Remove from the oven and let cool on a wire rack.

Cocoa Brownies

MAKES 16 BROWNIES

Gourmet recipes are sometimes difficult to make vegan, but Chef Ali and Mayim are glad they put the work into these brownies. Some have declared them the "best brownies ever" and we tend to agree. Sticky, chewy, and very gooey, these are amazing on their own, but we like them as the basis for a vegan brownie sundae, with vegan ice cream, whipped cream, and a cherry on top.

Nonstick cooking spray
10 tablespoons vegan margarine, cut into 1-inch pieces
1¼ cups sugar
¾ cup natural unsweetened cocoa powder
1 teaspoon vanilla extract
¼ teaspoon salt
½ cup applesauce
⅓ cup plus 1 tablespoon unbleached all-purpose flour
1 cup chopped walnuts

1. Position the rack in bottom third of oven and preheat to 325°F. Line an 8-inch baking pan with aluminum foil, pressing the foil firmly against the pan sides and leaving a 2-inch overhang. Coat the foil with nonstick cooking spray.
2. In a medium saucepan over medium heat, melt the margarine for about 2 minutes, stirring constantly. Remove from the heat and immediately add the sugar, cocoa powder, 2 teaspoons of water, and the vanilla and salt. Stir to blend. Let cool for 5 minutes (the mixture will still be hot).
3. Add the applesauce and mix well. When it looks thick, after about 1 minute, add the flour and stir until blended. Beat vigorously for 60 strokes. Stir in the nuts. Transfer the batter to the prepared pan.
4. Bake the brownies until a toothpick inserted into the center comes out almost clean (with a few moist crumbs attached), about 35 minutes. Let cool in the pan on a wire rack for another 30 minutes. Using the foil overhang, gently lift the brownies from the pan. Cut into 16 squares.

Dark Chocolate Peanut Butter Pie

Three ingredients, one prepared piecrust: that's it. Mayim's friend Joey told her about this recipe, and it has become a standard in her house and in the homes of everyone she has passed it on to. It's simple to make and tastes like a professional peanut butter cup. Top it with sliced bananas, decorate it with vegan whipped cream, or just eat it straight out of the pie dish. However you enjoy it, you will see why we just can't get enough of this pie.

2 cups vegan dark chocolate chips
1½ cups creamy peanut butter
1 (13.5-ounce) can coconut milk
Prepared vegan piecrust, preferably graham cracker

1. Melt the chocolate chips in a glass bowl in the microwave, stirring twice, about 3 minutes. Stir until the chocolate is completely melted. Stir in the peanut butter and coconut milk until combined.
2. Pour into the prepared piecrust and refrigerate until firm, about 2 hours.

Halloween Candy Bark

MAKES ABOUT 2 POUNDS, OR THIRTY 2-INCH PIECES BARK

Even vegans need candy bark once in a while, right? This veganized template of candy bark is so much fun. To make this bark, Mayim seeks out vegan versions of popular candy bars everywhere she goes, including kosher candy stores or markets, where nondairy candy is readily available. Once you get the chocolate base, improvise with whatever candy you like. Look for at least three different types for the most appeal. This is a gorgeous and delicious bark for Halloween or any time of year!

1 (24-ounce) bag vegan chocolate chips

6 (2- to 3-ounce) vegan chocolate bars, cut into ¾- to 1-inch pieces

8 medium-size vegan peanut butter cups, each cut into 8 wedges

3 ounces vegan white chocolate

½ cup sweetened or candied peanuts

1 cup yellow and orange vegan chocolate-covered peanuts (basically, these are vegan peanut M&M's, often available at kosher markets)

1. Line a baking sheet with aluminum foil.
2. Fill a medium pot halfway with water and bring to a boil. Place the chocolate chips in a metal bowl and place the bowl over the boiling water. Stir over low heat until melted and warm to the touch, about 8 minutes. Alternatively, melt in a microwave, stirring every minute to prevent burning. Pour the chocolate onto the prepared baking sheet and, using a spatula, spread out into a 12 × 10-inch rectangle about ¼ inch thick. Sprinkle with chocolate bar pieces and peanut butter cup wedges, making sure all the pieces touch the melted chocolate, to adhere.
3. Place the white chocolate in a separate metal bowl over a pot of boiling water.. Stir constantly over very low heat until the chocolate is melted and warm to the touch, about 8 minutes. Remove from the heat. Use a spoon to pour zigzag lines over the bark. Scatter the sweetened peanuts and chocolate-covered peanuts over the top, making sure everything touches melted chocolate.

4. Refrigerate the bark until cold and firm, about 30 minutes. Slide the bark onto a work surface and peel off the foil. Break the bark into irregular pieces about 2 inches wide.

NOTE: *Store in an airtight container for up to 4 days, if it lasts that long without being eaten!*

Candy Cane Winter Bark

MAKES ABOUT TWELVE 2-INCH PIECES BARK

We can't imagine the winter holidays without peppermint bark. Here's a vegan version that is easy to make and so easy to love.

12 ounces vegan semisweet chocolate chips
¼ cup plain, unsweetened soy milk
10 candy canes, chopped into small pieces

1. Line a baking sheet with parchment paper.
2. In the top of a double boiler, or in a medium stainless-steel bowl set over a pot of gently simmering water, melt the chocolate with the soy milk until smooth. Pour onto the prepared baking sheet, and using a spatula, spread the chocolate mixture evenly across the whole pan. Sprinkle with the candy canes pieces.
3. Refrigerate for 3 hours, until firm. Slide the bark onto a work surface and peel off the parchment paper. Break the bark into irregular pieces about 2 inches wide.

NOTE: *Store in an airtight container for up to 4 days.*

Pecan Pie Truffles

MAKES 24 TRUFFLES

Every Thanksgiving, Mayim makes these for her girlfriends, and every Thanksgiving, everyone wonders why she doesn't make them every week. With or without the bourbon, these truffles are rich and tasty.

2 ½ cups pecans, toasted and finely chopped
1 cup vegan graham cracker crumbs
1 cup brown sugar
½ teaspoon salt
2 tablespoons maple syrup
¼ cup bourbon
1 teaspoon vanilla extract
7 ounces vegan dark chocolate

1. On a rimmed baking sheet, toast the chopped pecans in a 325°F oven for 8 to 10 minutes, watching them closely, until they start to darken. You can also use a toaster oven or sauté them without oil in a small pan until they brown and become fragrant, about 5 minutes. Remove from the heat and set aside.
2. In a medium bowl, stir together the toasted pecans, graham cracker crumbs, brown sugar, and salt until well combined. Add the maple syrup, bourbon, and vanilla, stirring thoroughly. Use your hands to make sure the mixture becomes fully incorporated.
3. Form the candy into 24 walnut-size balls. Place them on a baking sheet and freeze for 2 hours.
4. In the top of a double boiler, or in a medium stainless-steel bowl set over a pot of gently simmering water, melt the chocolate. Line a baking sheet with parchment paper or a Silpat. Dip the frozen balls into the melted chocolate, and place on the prepared baking sheet. Let the truffles sit for 15 minutes, or until firm.

NOTE: *Store at room temperature in an airtight container, for up to 1 week.*

Chocolate, Fruit, and Nut Clusters

MAKES ABOUT 18 CLUSTERS

These clusters call for just a few ingredients and they are a hit every time. The chocolate is very rich, so keep the clusters small so that they are not overpowering.

½ cup vegan semisweet chocolate chips or baking chocolate bar, chopped
½ cup vegan bittersweet chocolate chips
½ cup dried cranberries
½ cup pecans, coarsely chopped and toasted

1. Using a rimmed baking sheet, toast the chopped pecans for 8 to 10 minutes, watching closely. You could also use a toaster oven until the pecans start to darken, or sauté without oil in a small pan until they brown and become fragrant, about 5 minutes. Remove and set aside.
2. Fill a medium pot halfway with water and bring to a boil. Place the chocolate chips in a metal bowl and place the bowl over the boiling water. Stir over low heat until melted and warm to the touch, about 8 minutes. Alternatively, melt in a microwave, stirring every minute to prevent burning.
3. Stir in the cranberries and toasted pecans. Immediately drop by level tablespoonfuls onto a waxed paper–lined baking sheet, placing about 1 inch apart so they are not touching. Refrigerate until the chocolate is set, about 30 minutes.

NOTE: *Clusters will keep in the refrigerator up to 5 days.*

Mandel Brodt

Eastern Europeans refer to **mandel brodt** *(almond bread) as "Jewish biscotti." Indeed, this crunchy cookie is baked twice and tastes best dunked in a cup of coffee.*

Nonstick cooking spray
4 tablespoons (½ stick) vegan margarine
3 cups all-purpose flour
1 cup sugar
1 teaspoon baking powder
1 teaspoon vanilla extract
¾ cup walnuts, chopped
Egg replacer equivalent of 3 eggs
1 teaspoon ground cinnamon (optional)

1. Preheat the oven to 350°F. Spray a baking sheet with cooking spray.
2. In a large bowl, mix all the ingredients to form a thick dough. Divide the dough in half. Place on the prepared baking sheet and shape into two loaves.
3. Bake for 30 minutes.
4. Remove from the oven and carefully cut the loaves into ½-inch slices. Lay the slices on their side on another pan and bake for 5 to 10 minutes more, until starting to harden at the edges.

CHOCOLATE VARIATION: Divide the dough in half. To one of the halves, add 3 tablespoons of natural unsweetened cocoa powder, 4 tablespoons of sugar, and 1 tablespoon of oil. Form into a loaf and bake as indicated.

Plum and Walnut Crisp

SERVES 6

This fruit crisp is a summer tradition for Mayim's family. Her sons' Grandma has a plum tree, and she always brings pounds and pounds of plums with her to visit in the summer. Mayim makes the crisp when the plums are ripe and freezes it for later reheating and enjoying in the fall.

TOPPING
½ cup all-purpose flour
½ cup packed light brown sugar
½ teaspoon ground cinnamon
¼ teaspoon ground ginger
¼ teaspoon salt
Pinch of ground nutmeg
6 tablespoons chilled unsalted vegan margarine, cut into ½-inch cubes
1 cup walnuts, coarsely chopped

FILLING
2½ pounds plums, quartered and pitted (see Kitchen Tip)
½ cup sugar
1 tablespoon cornstarch
1 teaspoon vanilla extract

1. To make the topping, combine the flour, brown sugar, cinnamon, ginger, salt, and nutmeg in large bowl. Add the margarine and rub it in with your fingertips until small, moist clumps form. Mix in the walnuts. Cover and refrigerate 20 minutes.
2. Preheat the oven to 400°F.
3. To make the filling, toss the plums, sugar, cornstarch, and vanilla in a large bowl to combine. Let stand until the sugar dissolves, tossing occasionally, about 5 minutes.
4. Transfer the filling to an 11 × 7-inch baking dish. Sprinkle the topping over the filling. Bake until the topping is dark golden brown and crisp and the filling

is bubbling, about 40 minutes. Transfer the pan to a wire rack and let cool for 30 minutes.

NOTE: *Serve this crisp very warm, with a pint of vegan vanilla ice cream. You can give it a "homemade" touch by mixing in ¼ cup of chopped crystallized ginger. Microwave the ice cream on low for 5-second intervals, just until slightly softened. Place in medium bowl and mix in the ginger. Cover and freeze until firm.*

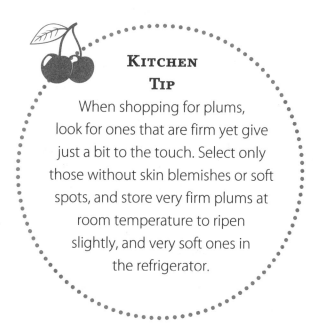

KITCHEN TIP

When shopping for plums, look for ones that are firm yet give just a bit to the touch. Select only those without skin blemishes or soft spots, and store very firm plums at room temperature to ripen slightly, and very soft ones in the refrigerator.

No-Fail Vanilla Cake

SERVES 8 TO 10

Mayim's friend Denise (the photographer for this book) introduced this cake to their circle of moms. This light and not-too-sweet cake is great for cupcakes, too, and can be frosted however you choose. It's great with the CHOCOLATE FROSTING *in the* CHOCOLATE FUDGE CAKE *recipe on* PAGE 194.

Nonstick cooking spray
2 cups unbleached white flour
1½ teaspoons baking powder
½ teaspoon baking soda
½ teaspoon sea salt
¼ cup canola oil
¾ cup plus 2 tablespoons maple syrup
¾ cup rice or soy milk
2 teaspoons cider vinegar
3 tablespoons vanilla extract

1. Preheat the oven to 350°F. Spray two 8-inch round cake pans with cooking spray and line the bottoms with parchment paper.
2. Sift the flours, baking powder, baking soda, and sea salt into a medium bowl and stir with a whisk to mix.
3. Whisk the oil, maple syrup, nondairy milk, vinegar, and vanilla in a medium bowl until foamy. Pour into the dry ingredients and mix until the batter is smooth.
4. Pour the batter into the pans, dividing it evenly. Level the tops by gently rotating the pans. Tap the pans lightly on the counter to eliminate air bubbles.
5. Bake the cakes for 20 to 25 minutes on the center rack of the oven, or until the cake is golden brown and springs back at its center when touched lightly. A toothpick inserted into the center should come out almost clean with a few moist crumbs attached.

6. Remove the cakes from the oven and place the pans on wire racks. Let the cakes cool in their pans for 10 minutes, then run a knife around the pan sides to loosen the cakes. Turn the layers out of the pans directly onto a wire rack, to finish cooling.

7. When cool, enclose each layer tightly in plastic wrap. Refrigerate until the layers are cold, about 1 hour, before filling and frosting, or wrap in foil for longer storage.

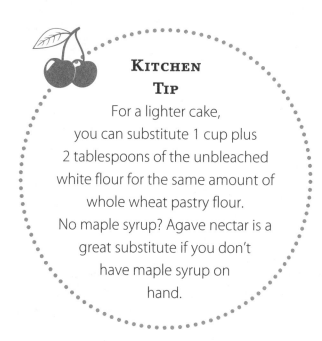

KITCHEN TIP

For a lighter cake, you can substitute 1 cup plus 2 tablespoons of the unbleached white flour for the same amount of whole wheat pastry flour.
No maple syrup? Agave nectar is a great substitute if you don't have maple syrup on hand.

Chocolate Fudge Cake

SERVES 12

Here is an easy and basic frosted chocolate cake that will work every time. Use this as the basis for birthday cakes, cupcakes, or any dessert requiring a moist and chocolaty base.

CHOCOLATE CAKE

3 cups all-purpose flour

2 cups sugar

6 tablespoons natural unsweetened cocoa powder

1 teaspoon salt

2 teaspoons baking soda

2 cups warm water

¾ cup vegetable oil

1 tablespoon white vinegar

2 teaspoons vanilla extract

CHOCOLATE FROSTING

1 (10-ounce) package vegan chocolate chips

1 (12.3-ounce) package silken extra-firm tofu

3 tablespoons maple syrup or agave nectar

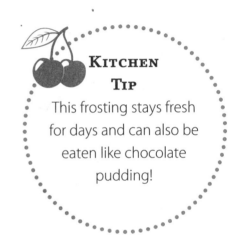

KITCHEN TIP

This frosting stays fresh for days and can also be eaten like chocolate pudding!

1. Preheat the oven to 350°F. Sift the flour, sugar, cocoa powder, salt, and baking soda together into a bowl.

2. Add the warm water, oil, vinegar, and vanilla. Beat until smooth, 2 to 3 minutes.

3. Bake in a 9 × 13-inch pan for 30 to 40 minutes, until a toothpick inserted into the center comes out almost clean (with a few moist crumbs attached). Let cool in the pan and remove from the pan.

4. To make the frosting: In the top of a double boiler, or in a medium stainless-steel bowl set over a pot of gently simmering water, melt the chocolate until smooth. Place the tofu and maple syrup in a blender and add the melted chocolate. Blend until mixed. Cover and refrigerate overnight. Spread on top of the cake, using the back of a spoon or a cake froster.

Rugelach

MAKES 24 RUGELACH

One of the best-known Jewish pastries, rugelach are flaky cookies with a variety of fill-ings. They're rolled up like tiny croissants and baked until golden. This recipe calls for a filling of cinnamon, sugar, and nuts, but you can also fill them with jam or tiny vegan chocolate chips.

DOUGH

2 cups all-purpose flour

½ teaspoon salt

12 tablespoons (1½ sticks) vegan margarine, chilled, plus 4 tablespoons (½ stick), melted

2 tablespoons white vinegar

1 cup cold water

1 cup sugar

2 teaspoons ground cinnamon

½ cup nuts, chopped (optional)

1. Sift the flour and salt together in a large bowl. Cut in the chilled margarine until the flour is crumbly as it is starting to be incorporated into the margarine, but not until it feels or looks smooth. Add the vinegar to the cold water and stir. Sprinkle a little at a time into the flour mixture. Work with your fingers or a fork until the dough just comes together. The dough should not be sticky.

2. Shape the dough into a ball and place in a resealable plastic bag. Refrigerate for 2 hours.

3. Preheat the oven to 425°F. Divide the dough into eight equal portions and form into 8 balls. Roll each ball into a 7-inch-diameter circle. Brush with the melted margarine. Sprinkle with the sugar, nuts, and cinnamon. Cut each circle in half and then into quarters. Roll each wedge from the outside edge toward the center, like a croissant.

4. Bake the rugelach on a baking sheet for 15 minutes, spaced 1 inch apart, then lower the heat to 375°F and bake for another 10 to 15 minutes, until starting to turn golden.

Sufganiyot

Chanukah is a Jewish winter holiday celebrating a military battle and a miracle of oil over two thousand years ago. Jews eat foods fried in oil during this holiday, and **sufganiyot** *(doughnuts) are enjoyed for the entire eight-day holiday. This veganized recipe makes outrageously light and delicious doughnuts, which can be filled with jam but are delectable when simply sprinkled with confectioners' sugar. These doughnuts are best enjoyed the day you make them. Make sure to drain them well before serving.*

1 (0.25-ounce) envelope active dry yeast

½ cup sugar

1 cup plus 2 tablespoons warm soy, rice, or almond milk (about 110°F)

3½ cups all-purpose flour, plus more for dusting

1¼ teaspoons coarse salt

Egg replacer equivalent of 2 eggs

3 tablespoons unsalted vegan margarine, melted and cooled

Nonstick cooking spray

About 6 cups vegetable oil, for frying

Confectioners' sugar, for sprinkling

About 2 cups raspberry jam (optional)

1. Combine the yeast, sugar and 1 cup of the warm nondairy milk in a small bowl and let stand until foamy, about 8 minutes.

2. Whisk together the flour and salt in a bowl. Add the yeast mixture, egg replacer, and margarine, and beat until the dough is soft but not sticky, about 3 minutes.

3. On a lightly floured surface, knead the dough until smooth and elastic, 3 to 4 minutes. Transfer the dough to a medium bowl coated with nonstick cooking spray, and cover loosely with plastic wrap. Let rise in a warm, draft-free place until doubled in size, about 1½ hours.

4. Punch down the dough. On a lightly floured surface, knead the dough a few times, and roll out to ¼ inch thick. Cover with a clean dish towel, and let rest for 5 minutes.

5. Using a 2-inch-diameter cookie cutter, cut out rounds and transfer to a lightly floured baking sheet. Reroll the scraps, and cut out the remaining dough. Cover the rounds with a clean dish towel and let rise slightly in a warm, draft-free place for 20 minutes.

6. Meanwhile, heat the oil in a large, heavy-bottomed pot until it reaches 375°F. Place a wire rack on top of parchment paper or on a baking sheet, and line with paper towels or brown paper bags. Working in batches of four or five, add the doughnuts to the hot oil and fry, turning once, until golden and puffed, about 1 minute per side. Using a slotted spoon, place the doughnuts on the paper towels to cool. Sprinkle with confectioners' sugar.

VARIATION: For jam-filled doughnuts, spoon jam into a pastry bag fitted with a plain ⅜-inch tip. Pierce a hole in the side of a doughnut with the tip, and squeeze in jam to fill (filled doughnut will feel heavy).

NOTE: *These doughnuts are best when served immediately, but they can be stored in air-tight containers overnight.*

Hamantaschen

MAKES 4 DOZEN HAMANTASCHEN

The Jewish holiday of Purim is celebrated with ritual foods such as these three-sided cookies. Called "Haman's Pockets," they are named for the villain of the Purim story, which occurred in Persia in the fourth century BCE. The dough is sweet and dense, and any variety of fillings will work well with the versatile dough. Mayim and her mom make a "mishmash" filling from 1 cup of any jam with 2 tablespoons of melted vegan chocolate chips and 1 tablespoon of chopped almonds or walnuts. If you want suggestions for more traditional fillings, see below.

Canola cooking spray
1 cup sugar
½ cup oil
8 tablespoons (1 stick) vegan margarine
Egg replacer equivalent of 3 eggs
½ cup orange juice, freshly squeezed if possible
4 cups all-purpose flour
1 to 2 teaspoons baking powder
1 teaspoon salt

1. Preheat the oven to 350°F and grease a baking sheet.
2. Cream sugar, oil, and margarine in a large bowl. Add the egg replacer and orange juice, mixing well. Add the flour, baking powder, and salt and mix well. The dough will be smooth, with all ingredients well incorporated.
3. On a floured surface, roll out the dough to about ⅛ inch thick. Flour the rim of a glass and cut out circles. Place about 2 teaspoons of your filling of choice in the middle of each circle.
4. To shape the triangular hamantaschen, pinch together the top and left side of the circle toward the middle. Do the same with the top and right side of the circle. Join the sides together. Bake on the prepared baking sheet until slightly browned.

Variations: Other ideas for fillings:

- Any flavor of jam
- Pitted and chopped dates
- Lekvar (cooked prune concentrate)
- Poppy-seed paste

METRIC CONVERSIONS

The recipes in this book have not been tested with metric measurements, so some variations might occur.

Remember that the weight of dry ingredients varies according to the volume or density factor: 1 cup of flour weighs far less than 1 cup of sugar, and 1 tablespoon doesn't necessarily hold 3 teaspoons.

 ### General Formulas for Metric Conversion

Ounces to grams	$\Rightarrow$ ounces × 28.35 = grams
Grams to ounces	$\Rightarrow$ grams × 0.035 = ounces
Pounds to grams	$\Rightarrow$ pounds × 453.5 = grams
Pounds to kilograms	$\Rightarrow$ pounds × 0.45 = kilograms
Cups to liters	$\Rightarrow$ cups × 0.24 = liters
Fahrenheit to Celsius	$\Rightarrow$ (°F − 32) × 5 ÷ 9 = °C
Celsius to Fahrenheit	$\Rightarrow$ (°C × 9) ÷ 5 + 32 = °F

Linear Measurements

½ inch = 1½ cm
1 inch = 2½ cm
6 inches = 15 cm
8 inches = 20 cm
10 inches = 25 cm
12 inches = 30 cm
20 inches = 50 cm

 ### Oven Temperature Equivalents, Fahrenheit (F) and Celsius (C)

100°F = 38°C
200°F = 95°C
250°F = 120°C
300°F = 150°C
350°F = 180°C
400°F = 205°C
450°F = 230°C

 ### Weight (Mass) Measurements

1 ounce = 30 grams
2 ounces = 55 grams
3 ounces = 85 grams
4 ounces = ¼ pound = 125 grams
8 ounces = ½ pound = 240 grams
12 ounces = ¾ pound = 375 grams
16 ounces = 1 pound = 454 grams

Volume (Dry) Measurements

¼ teaspoon = 1 milliliter
½ teaspoon = 2 milliliters
¾ teaspoon = 4 milliliters
1 teaspoon = 5 milliliters
1 tablespoon = 15 milliliters
¼ cup = 59 milliliters
⅓ cup = 79 milliliters
½ cup = 118 milliliters
⅔ cup = 158 milliliters
¾ cup = 177 milliliters
1 cup = 225 milliliters
4 cups or 1 quart = 1 liter
½ gallon = 2 liters
1 gallon = 4 liters

Volume (Liquid) Measurements

1 teaspoon = ⅙ fluid ounce = 5 milliliters
1 tablespoon = ½ fluid ounce = 15 milliliters
2 tablespoons = 1 fluid ounce = 30 milliliters
¼ cup = 2 fluid ounces = 60 milliliters
⅓ cup = 2 ⅔ fluid ounces = 79 milliliters
½ cup = 4 fluid ounces = 118 milliliters
1 cup or ½ pint = 8 fluid ounces = 250 milliliters
2 cups or 1 pint = 16 fluid ounces = 500 milliliters
4 cups or 1 quart = 32 fluid ounces = 1,000 milliliters
1 gallon = 4 liters

Resources

Books

Cookbooks

Barnard, Tanya, and Sarah Kramer. *How It All Vegan!: Irresistible Recipes for an Animal-Free Diet*. Arsenal Pulp Press, 2002.

> This is the "punk rock" vegan resource and cookbook that many find irresistible, largely because of the fresh and hip perspective the authors present. Barnard and Kramer offer great recipes, substitution ideas for new vegans, and a really fun presentation.

Gentry, Ann. *The Real Food Daily Cookbook: Really Fresh, Really Good, Really Vegetarian*. Ten Speed Press, 2005.

> The first gourmet vegan restaurant in Los Angeles is well known for a reason: the food is spectacular, it contains no refined sugar, and the emphasis is on clean, healthy, and delicious. The RFD cookbook allows you to create its recipes in your home with great success and it's a wonderful basic cookbook for any kitchen.

Moskowitz, Isa Chandra, and Terry Hope Romero. *Veganomicon: The Ultimate Vegan Cookbook*. Da Capo Lifelong Books, 2007.

> These two vegan chefs are among the best out there. This large, user-friendly cookbook features outstanding and easy-to-make recipes, including soy-free and gluten-free recipes as well.

Patrick-Goudreau, Colleen. *The Joy of Vegan Baking: The Compassionate Cooks' Traditional Treats and Sinful Sweets*. Fair Winds Press, 2006.

> Being vegan doesn't mean giving up your favorite cookies, cakes, pies, and pastries. This is the book that helps you re-create all of your favorites, only vegan!

Ronnen, Tal. *The Conscious Cook: Delicious Meatless Recipes That Will Change the Way You Eat*. William Morrow Cookbooks, 2009.

> Perhaps known best for being Oprah Winfrey's, Ellen DeGeneres's, and Portia de Rossi's chef, Tal Ronnen creates satisfying recipes for the most discriminating foodie.

Silverstone, Alicia. *The Kind Diet: A Simple Guide to Feeling Great, Losing Weight, and Saving the Planet.* Rodale Books, 2009.

Actress Alicia Silverstone changed the public face of veganism with this book, emphasizing ethics and health as reasons to go vegan. Some of the recipes are complicated and require some unusual ingredients, but the text is thorough and the recipe for peanut butter cups is one you can't live without!

Tucker, Eric. *The Artful Vegan: Fresh Flavors from the Millennium Restaurant.* Ten Speed Press, 2003.

This is the cookbook of San Francisco's famous gourmet Millennium Restaurant. The book features spectacular global vegan cuisine and most recipes are cholesterol and oil-free as well.

Nutrition & Health

Campbell, T. Colin, and Thomas M. Campbell II. *The China Study: The Most Comprehensive Study of Nutrition Ever Conducted and the Startling Implications for Diet, Weight Loss, and Long-term Health.* Dallas, TX: Benbella Books, 2006.

This quintessential apolitical book is based on large-scale long-term research into the diet and lifestyle of thousands of individuals. It shows the connection between nutrition and heart disease, diabetes, and cancer and also addresses the nutritional complexity of lobbies and the role of the government

and popular scientists in the discussion of a plant-based diet.

Davis, Brenda, and Vesanto Melina. *Becoming Vegan: The Complete Guide to Adopting a Healthy Plant-Based Diet.* Book Publishing Company, 2000.

As registered dietitians, Davis and Melina present a sound and friendly approach to understanding veganism. From health benefits to nutritional assessments to making the transition, this is a wonderful industry standard for transitioning to a plant-based lifestyle.

Esselstyn, Caldwell B., Jr. *Prevent and Reverse Heart Disease: The Revolutionary, Scientifically Proven, Nutrition-Based Cure.* Avery Trade, 2008.

One of the foremost and earliest plant-based medical advocates, Dr. Esselstyn is a surgeon and clinician who challenges conventional cardiology in this groundbreaking book. This book explores the results of his twenty-year nutritional study and argues that a plant-based, oil-free diet can prevent and stop the progression of heart disease, and also reverse its effects.

Lappé, Frances Moore. *Diet for a Small Planet.* Ballantine Books, 1991.

Frances Moore Lappé is a trailblazer in the plant-based world. This remarkable book focuses on a plant-based lifestyle as an act of social, environmental, and economic transformation on a personal and global scale.

Ornish, Dean. *Dr. Dean Ornish's Program for Reversing Heart Disease: The Only System Scientifically Proven to Reverse Heart Disease Without Drugs or Surgery.* Ivy Books, 1995.

This groundbreaking book was the first to offer documented proof by a clinician that heart disease can be halted and even reversed by changing your lifestyle. This book represents the intersection of modern medicine and the vegan diet in a very powerful way.

Robbins, John. *Diet for a New America: How Your Food Choices Affect Your Health, Happiness, and the Future of Life on Earth.* HJ Kramer/New World Library, 2012.

Diet for a New America is considered to be one of the most important books about the astounding moral, economic, and emotional price we pay for the "American diet." It is a classic and this new edition is even more powerful and relevant than when it was first published.

Ethics/Lifestyle

Barnounin, Kim, and Rory Freedman. *Skinny Bitch*, Running Press, 2005.

Although the title of this book indicates a motivation of being thin, this book launched a plant-based and whole foods–based revolution, particularly among women unfamiliar with the benefits of a vegan lifestyle before.

Foer, Jonathan Safran. *Eating Animals*. Back Bay Books, 2009.

This is the book that made Mayim 100 percent vegan. Safran Foer, a respected novelist, writes about his personal journey into researching factory farming as he awaited the birth of his first child, and the horrifying and powerful conclusions he came to after his research. This is a beautifully and passionately written exposé into the truth behind the animal food industry and the decisions we make when we confront them.

Scully, Matthew. *Dominion: The Power of Man, the Suffering of Animals, and the Call to Mercy*. St. Martin's Griffin, 2003.

Scully is a journalist and former speechwriter for President George W. Bush. His book on animal welfare does not insist upon equal "rights" for animals but argues for treating them with respect. Scully personally investigates several animal industries and shows the logical and political inconsistencies used to defend them. This is a very powerful book, and a very philosophically sound one as well.

Websites

Recipes

http://www.lukasvolger.com—Known primarily for his veggie burger recipes, Lukas Volger is a go-to for hearty whole foods–based vegan cuisine.

http://www.veganyumyum.com—Lauren Ulm is a pioneer of vegan gourmet food. Her recipes are known to be delicious, presented beautifully, and appealing to vegans and nonvegans alike.

http://www.yumuniverse.com—Heather Crosby is a recipe developer for plant-based, gluten-free, wheat-free, dairy-free, and meat-free foods and is a T. Colin Campbell Foundation certified plant-based nutrition coach. Yum Universe contains recipes, meal plans, and excellent resources for a plant-based lifestyle.

Lifestyle

http://www.happycow.net—HappyCow is a nonprofit online community that assists travelers in finding vegan, vegetarian, and healthy food wherever they go.

http://www.kriscarr.com—This is the fascinating and informative website of a *New York Times* best-selling author, wellness activist, and cancer survivor.

http://www.veganessentials.com—This all-inclusive website has links and resources for everything from where to get vegan beef jerky to vitamins to shoes to perfume. It's one of the best websites for all things vegan.

http://www.vegfamily.com—*VegFamily* is an online vegan magazine with an emphasis on families and kids. Recipes, articles, opinions, and expert Q & A are standard features.

http://www.vegnews.com—The premier vegan lifestyle magazine, featuring vegan news, food and recipes, travel, and politics. It's read in over thirty-eight countries and is a fantastic resource for all things vegan.

http://www.vegsource.com—A comprehensive website including videos, book reviews, recipes, and news.

Health

http://www.drmcdougall.com—Excellent resources by a physician and nutrition expert who teaches and writes about better health through a plant-based diet.

http://www.zerotothree.org/child-development/health-nutrition/tips-and-tools-on-health-and.html. Website of Zero to Three.

This is an excellent national nonprofit organization dedicated to educating parents, practitioners, and the community about the critical first three years of development, concerning nutrition, neurodevelopment, and education.

Ethics

http://www.goveg.com—PETA is the largest animal rights organization in the world, with more than 3 million supporters and members. Its four areas of focus include factory farms, animal research, animals used for clothing, and the abuse of animals in the entertainment industry.

http://www.PCRM.org—PCRM leads the nation in reforming federal nutrition policies and groundbreaking research, including alternatives to animal research and testing. Some of the biggest names in medicine and nutrition serve on the advisory board and board of directors, including T. Colin Campbell, PhD, Caldwell B. Esselstyn, Jr., MD, Andrew Weil, MD, and Neal D. Barnard, MD.

Acknowledgments

Mayim Bialik

My maternal grandmother, Sura Perl, hailed from Muncach, where Hungarian cooking and baking was taken very seriously. She was a hard-working *baalabusta* and she taught my mother well how to cook with love. My paternal grandmother, Jennie, claimed, "I never used a spice in my life," thereby raising my father with a lot to look forward to in the kitchen when he married my mother. His self-described "child's palate" forced my mother to be creative and find ways to feed two children and a husband, all of whom had a "child's palate."

My mother was ahead of her time nutritionally, refusing in the 1970s to feed me cow's milk, sugary cereals, or more than a raw carrot and a rice cake as snacks for the first fifteen years of my life. Complain as I did then, I can now admit how much I appreciate the good groundwork she laid for my health and my diet. She always made meals attractive and orderly, even when life was chaotic and money was sparse. She, like my grandmothers before her, was exclusively responsible for making every single meal I ever ate, unless you count the "fruit face" or "vegetable face" my father made for me a few times a year. I am thrilled that my parents have embraced a vegetarian lifestyle since they have retired.

To my closest friends Adi Rubin and Kari Druyen. You both hail from fiery Sabra mothers whose kitchens were the social and emotional hub of your loving childhood homes. You are women who are proud of your cooking, comfortable in your kitchens, and gracefully show your families love with what you make and bake. *Todah rabah* for cooking for me and baking me challah when my hands could not.

To my sons' father, Michael, who hailed from a culinary background very different from my own. You were raised where everything had sour cream and extra butter and some part of a pig mixed in. Thank you for raising our children vegan. Many of the recipes in this book were inspired by your desires for the rich and "all-American" recipes of your childhood, minus the pig bits. Sushi Bowl? Genuis.

To Fancy Assistant Brandon, who hails from a part of the country where the word *vegan* is only whispered in hushed tones and where it means certain starvation and deprivation. Oh, Missouri: thank you for making Brandon curious and open-minded, food-wise! Thank you for your patience when I had none, your typing skills when my hands could not type, and your editorial comments when I asked for them and even when I didn't. I trust your opinions and value your hard work and dedication to my career and life very much and I am grateful for your participation with this book especially.

To Dr. Jay Gordon, our pediatrician and my coauthor. Your support of a vegan lifestyle has saved the heart and body of countless children and families and your voice is a tremendously important part of this book. Thank you and Lorri Horn for your hard work and dedication!

To Anthony Mattero at Foundry Media, my book agent, for believing in this book's message, meaning, and tastiness. You have steered us through so many challenges so bravely. And thank you for marrying a dietician because without Lindsey, I would not have had the confidence to believe this book had legitimacy in the world of diet and nutrition.

To Renée Sedliar for taking on this book with excitement, sincerity, and a true desire to present attractive and accessible plant-based eating. This has been a wonderful journey and I am so very grateful to you for helping make this a reality. You are awesome.

My Kveller.com fans were the inspiration for this book, as they demanded to know how on earth I managed to celebrate all of those Jewish holidays without eggs, dairy, or meat! Well, Kveller gang: here you go!

To Chef Alison Cruddas, the fiery ginger-haired, tattooed goddess whose recipes filled in the blanks. Alison, your sense of humor and your vegan wisdom have inspired me for years. Working together to share these recipes has been so gratifying. I am proud to have your hands on my recipes, and I am so grateful for the ones you added. What a delicious and satisfying partnership we have made together!

To Denise Herrick Borchert. You were the one to inspire and help me to go 100 percent vegan, and I thank you for being the photographer for all of the beautiful pictures in this book. Being vegan is so much more than a way of eating for you; it's a way of life. I look to you for inspiration still. Thank you!

To our food stylist, Skylar. Your skills have made the food in this book look even better than I could have imagined! Thank you for helping us create pictures of these vegan recipes that are worth more than a thousand words.

To Jennifer Manley for fastidiously entering all of the recipes in this book with her chef's expertise and editorial wisdom. Thank you, Jen, for your loving time and hours of work!

To *VegNews* and PETA and all of the incredibly supportive and courageous men and women who believe in and advocate for veganism and animal rights all over the world. Thank you for urging me to keep putting myself out there even though people are still ignorant, judgmental, and sometimes downright mean. Having organizations dedicated to supporting a vegan lifestyle is what was missing for most of my life. I am so honored to have found you as an adult!

Thank you to my publicist and professional cheerleader extraordinaire, Heather Weiss at Much & House Public Relations. You are always 100 percent honest with me, you are helpful in everything I do, and you have been incredibly supportive of this book and my entire career and life. You are the engine that runs this crazy train, and this book is no exception. Maybe one day I'll make you a vegan, but until then, you are the best omnivore publicist and comrade that anyone could ask for. I am so grateful for you!

Thank you to the cooks I have admired and adapted recipes from. In particular, thank you to Chef Selma Brown Morrow: you were the first professional I ever met who got paid money to do what my mom had to do every day for free.

And to all of the nonvegans who have tasted food in my home and have both humored me and given me constructive criticism for years and years, most notably my parents, Michael's mother, Sherrie, his father, Bob, and his wife, Di-

ane: you all share in the authorship of this book. Thank you for giving us the room to raise your grandchildren vegan with (almost no) fighting about it.

Dr. Jay Gordon

If one wants to write a book, the most essential part of this endeavor is a smart, skilled writer to help an amateur doctor/author like me. Lorri Horn sat with me for hours and hours, turning my ideas, thoughts, and nutritional practices into coherent and readable paragraphs and chapters. She listened to my theories, experiences, and anecdotes and read and gathered research and data. When I wasn't paying attention, she asked my patients to let her tape record our checkups to capture my behind-the-door voice, and then did what others before her have not done: she got it onto paper. My name is on the cover and her heart and skill are inside the book. Thank you, Lorri.

Mayim Bialik is a courageous advocate for children and families. Important changes in the way we eat and the way we feed our children will come one parent and one child at a time. She's deservedly famous and respected for her acting and much more. And she's "using her powers for the forces of good!"

My wife, Meyera, makes the rest of my life coherent and fills it with love, intelligence, and meaning. She supports everything I do, except the dumb things, and even then she guides me toward getting back on track. We've been together for almost four decades. Tired yet?

Our daughter Simone is my brilliant, challenging hiking buddy four early mornings each week. She fits me in between her master's studies, time as a city commissioner and everything else. She calls me on my inconsistencies and focuses me on real life nutrition. Wonderful, sweetie, just wonderful!

I could not practice medicine the way I do without a fantastic staff to support me. Lisa Boehle, Tammi Burns, Stephanie Crespin, Jennifer Davidson, Holly Factor, Lucy Griffin, Ileana Hernandez, Amy Hollis, Beverly Kitz, Ranessa Loving, Sophia Dibs, Marci Tarle, and Breena Yeh help me give my patients the attention they deserve. They keep the office running smoothly and contribute to the caring atmosphere that is so important. Lorri Horn is my cowriter and COO.

Ileana Hernandez has managed our office and has had to knock on that same office door to get me moving for well over twenty years. Bryan Sanders helps me with all thinking technological and works to make my website visible. Cheryl Taylor is the world's number one breastfeeding expert; breastfeeding is the heart and foundation of great nutrition and Cheryl has helped tens of thousands of mothers and babies as the real power behind the website with my name on it, drjaygordon.com.

I work with three skilled caring doctors in my office, Linda Nussbaum, Jody Lappin, and Alessia Gottlieb. I trust them and love my professional relationship and friendship with these excellent physicians.

Anthony Mattero is the most patient and best book agent ever.

Children, I really do eat a salad as big as my head at dinner every night.

Index